T0245211

Abnormal Female Puberty

Heather L. Appelbaum
Editor

Abnormal Female Puberty

A Clinical Casebook

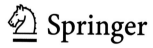 Springer

Editor
Heather L. Appelbaum, MD
Department of Obstetrics and Gynecology
Hofstra Northwell School of Medicine
New York, USA

ISBN 978-3-319-27223-8   ISBN 978-3-319-27225-2   (eBook)
DOI 10.1007/978-3-319-27225-2

Library of Congress Control Number: 2016932405

Springer Cham Heidelberg New York Dordrecht London
© Springer International Publishing Switzerland 2016

Printed on acid-free paper

Springer International Publishing AG Switzerland is part of Springer Science+Business Media (www.springer.com)

Preface

Female pubertal development requires coordination of the hypothalamus, pituitary, and ovaries and an appropriate outflow tract to allow for menstrual egress. The balance that is essential for adequate pubertal progress is delicate, requiring the appropriate hormonal and metabolic milieu for development. The hormonal axis may be influenced by intrinsic factors or exogenous exposures which can disrupt the normal process, manifesting in early or delayed signs of reaching specific pubertal milestones. The goal of *Abnormal Female Puberty: A Clinical Casebook* is to provide the practicing gynecologist, endocrinologist, pediatrician, adolescent medicine specialist, or reproductive endocrinologist with a concise volume that illustrates the tools required to treat both simple and complex pubertal problems. It provides a framework for understanding how to evaluate, diagnose, and manage a myriad of female pubertal disorders.

Chapter topics were chosen to cover the most pertinent and prevalent areas of abnormal pubertal development that a practitioner may encounter. Each chapter is formatted such that the reader can identify a problem and gain additional understanding of the fundamentals that relate to the disorder as well as appropriate treatment strategies. The chapters are organized to include examples related to the structural, hormonal, genetic, and environmental effects on pubertal development. The chapters include clinical pearls to help reinforce key points and learning objectives. Chapter authors were selected by the editor for their expertise in the field and asked to highlight real case examples to illustrate the focus of the respective chapters. The case book is a practical handbook that addresses various scenarios relating to abnormal pubertal development with the intention that the book can be used as a reference companion for further understanding focused clinical scenarios or used as an overview of abnormal female pubertal development.

I hope that this casebook becomes a frequently referenced guide for practicing physicians as well as allied health professionals, residents, fellows, or students who are interested in a greater appreciation of the factors that influence female pubertal development.

NY, USA   Heather L. Appelbaum, MD

Contents

1 Congenital Anomalies and Abnormal Pubertal Development 1
Heather L. Appelbaum and Amy Vallerie

2 Precocious Puberty 23
Jason Klein and Patricia M. Vuguin

3 Constitutional Delay of Growth and Puberty 47
M. Tracy Bekx and Ellen Lancon Connor

4 Premature Ovarian Failure 67
Amit Lahoti, Lakha Prasannan,
and Phyllis W. Speiser

5 Endocrine Disorders and Delayed Puberty 87
Allison Bauman, Laura Novello, and Paula Kreitzer

6 Androgenic Disorders and Abnormal Pubertal Development 109
Phyllis W. Speiser

7 Impact of Obesity on Female Puberty 127
Khalida Itriyeva and Ronald Feinstein

8 Anorexia Nervosa in the Young Female Adolescent 151
Martin Fisher and Alexis Santiago

**9   The Female Athlete Triad and Abnormal
      Pubertal Development** 175
      Maria C. Monge

**10   Celiac Disease and Abnormal Pubertal
      Development** 207
      Toni Webster and Michael Pettei

**11   Ovarian Neoplasms and Abnormal Pubertal
      Development** 225
      Jill S. Whyte

**12   Survivors of Childhood Cancer
      and Cancer Treatments** 241
      May-Tal Sauerbrun-Cutler, Christine Mullin,
      and Avner Hershlag

**13   Pharmacological and Environmental
      Effects on Pubertal Development** 261
      Veronica Gomez-Lobo

Index 271

Contributors

Heather L. Appelbaum, MD Division of Pediatric and Adolescent Gynecology, Cohen Children's Medical Center of NY/Long Island Jewish Medical Center, New Hyde Park, NY, USA

Department of Obstetrics and Gynecology, Hofstra Northwell School of Medicine, NY, USA

Allison Bauman, DO Division of Pediatric Endocrinology, Cohen Children's Medical Center of New York/Long Island Jewish Medical Center, Lake Success, NY, USA

M. Tracy Bekx, MD Division of Pediatric Endocrinology, University of Wisconsin, Madison, WI, USA

Ellen Lancon Connor, MD Division of Pediatric Endocrinology, University of Wisconsin, Madison, WI, USA

Ronald Feinstein, MD, FAAP Department of Adolescent Medicine, Cohen Children's Medical Center of New York, New Hyde Park, NY, USA

Martin Fisher, MD Division of Adolescent Medicine, Cohen Children's Medical Center, Northwell Health System, New Hyde Park, NY, USA

Hofstra Northwell School of Medicine, Hempstead, NY, USA

Veronica Gomez-Lobo, MD Washington Hospital Center/ Children's National Medical Center, Georgetown University, Washington, DC, USA

Avner Hershlag, MD Center for Human Reproduction, North Shore University Hospital—LIJ, Hofstra University School of Medicine, Manhasset, NY, USA

Khalida Itriyeva, MD Department of Adolescent Medicine, Cohen Children's Medical Center of New York, New Hyde Park, NY, USA

Jason Klein, MD Division of Pediatric Endocrinology, Cohen Children's Medical Center of NY, Lake Success, NY, USA

Hofstra Northwell School of Medicine, School of Medicine, Hempstead, NY, USA

Paula Kreitzer, MD Division of Pediatric Endocrinology, Cohen Children's Medical Center of New York/Long Island Jewish Medical Center, Lake Success, NY, USA

Hofstra Northwell School of Medicine, Hempstead, NY, USA

Amit Lahoti, MD Division of Pediatric Endocrinology, Le Bonheur Children's Hospital, University of Tennessee Health Science Center, Memphis, TN, USA

Maria C. Monge, MD Dell Children's Medical Center of Central Texas, University of Texas at Austin, Dell Medical School, Austin, TX, USA

Christine Mullin, MD Center for Human Reproduction, North Shore University Hospital—LIJ, Hofstra University School of Medicine, Manhasset, NY, USA

Laura Novello, MD Division of Pediatric Endocrinology, Cohen Children's Medical Center of New York/Long Island Jewish Medical Center, Lake Success, NY, USA

Michael Pettei, MD, PhD Division of Pediatric Gastroenterology and Nutrition, Cohen Children's Medical Center of NY/Long Island Jewish Medical Center, Lake Success, NY, USA

Hofstra Northwell School of Medicine, Hempstead, NY, USA

Lakha Prasannan, MD Department of Obstetrics and Gynecology, Northwell Health Systems, Hofstra Northwell School of Medicine, Hempstead, NY, USA

Alexis Santiago, MD Division of Adolescent Medicine, Cohen Children's Medical Center, Northwell Health System, New Hyde Park, NY, USA

May-Tal Sauerbrun-Cutler, MD Center for Human Reproduction, North Shore University Hospital—LIJ, Hofstra University School of Medicine, Manhasset, NY, USA

Phyllis W. Speiser, MD Division of Pediatric Endocrinology, Cohen Children's Medical Center of NY, Lake Success, NY, USA

Hofstra Northwell School of Medicine, Hempstead, NY, USA

Amy Vallerie, MD Obstetrics and Gynecology, Kaiser Permanente, Oakland, CA, USA

Patricia M. Vuguin, MSc, MD Hofstra Northwell School of Medicine, Hempstead, NY, USA

Toni Webster, DO, MSc Division of Pediatric Gastroenterology and Nutrition, Cohen Children's Medical Center of NY/Long Island Jewish Medical Center, Lake Success, NY, USA

Hofstra Northwell School of Medicine, Hempstead, NY, USA

Jill S. Whyte, MD Division of Gynecologic Oncology, North Shore University Hospital, Manhasset, NY, USA

Hofstra Northwell School of Medicine, Hempstead, NY, USA

Chapter 1
Congenital Anomalies and Abnormal Pubertal Development

Heather L. Appelbaum and Amy Vallerie

Abbreviations

17OHP	17-Hydroxyprogesterone
AIS	Androgen insensitivity
CAIS	Complete androgen insensitivity
DHEAS	DHEA-sulfate
DHT	Dihydrotestosterone
DSD	Disorders of sex development
FISH	Fluorescence in situ hybridization
FSH	Follicle-stimulating hormone
LH	Luteinizing hormone

H.L. Appelbaum, M.D. (✉)
Division of Pediatric and Adolescent Gynecology, Cohen Children's
Medical Center of NY/Long Island Jewish Medical Center, New Hyde
Park, NY 11040, USA

Department of Obstetrics and Gynecology, Hofstra Northwell School
of Medicine, 270-05, 76 th Ave, New Hyde Park, NY 11020, USA
e-mail: happelbaum@pedsgynecology.com

A. Vallerie, M.D.
Obstetrics and Gynecology, Kaiser Permanente, 3779 Piedmont Avenue,
Oakland, CA 94611, USA

© Springer International Publishing Switzerland 2016   1
H.L. Appelbaum (ed.), *Abnormal Female Puberty*,
DOI 10.1007/978-3-319-27225-2_1

MDA	Müllerian duct anomaly
MRKH	Mayer–Rokitnsky–Küster–Hauser
PAIS	Partial androgen insensitivity
SRY	Sex determining region Y

Introduction

Primary amenorrhea in girls is a frequent cause for referrals to the endocrinologist or gynecologist. Structural abnormalities of the reproductive tract account for approximately 22 % of cases of primary amenorrhea [1]. History and physical examination typically confirm normal progression of pubertal milestones, including normal thelarche, pubarche, and growth in girls who have not menstruated. In examining the patients, particular attention should be paid to breast development and Tanner staging, the presence of axillary and pubic hair, and careful inspection of the external genitalia and hymenal orifice. Laboratory determinations should be done to confirm normal gonadotropin and sex steroid hormone levels. Karyotype with FISH determination of the SRY gene is useful to appreciate if there is discordance between the phenotype and genotype of the individual [2, 3]. Imaging studies are essential in all cases to augment the physical findings and clarify the internal reproductive structures. This chapter will provide a case-based approach to appreciate the complexities of primary amenorrhea as a result of congenital anomalies of the reproductive tract. Surgical and nonsurgical treatment modalities will be discussed.

Müllerian Agenesis

Case Presentation

A 16-year-old female is referred for primary amenorrhea. Breast development began at age 11 years and she has had axillary and pubic hair since age 12. Her general health is good. She was diagnosed with scoliosis at age 9. She exercises regularly and eats a healthy, balanced diet. She is socially well adjusted. She is not sexually active and there is no family history of infertility.

On examination, her height 160 cm was and weight 59 kg; BMI was 21. Vital signs were normal. General habitus was normal for an adolescent girl. She had no acne or hirsutism. Pubertal status was Tanner stage 5 for breasts and pubic hair development and there was no clitoral enlargement. The hymen was annular and diminutive. Cotton-tipped applicator identified a 1 cm vaginal dimple. The urethra, perineum, and anus were normal.

Laboratory tests included normal thyroid functions, prolactin, luteinizing hormone (LH), follicle-stimulating hormone (FSH), estradiol, and DHEA-sulfate (DHEAS). Her early morning 17-hydroxyprogesterone (17OHP; tandem mass spectrometry assay) was normal and testosterone level was normal. Karyotype was 46, XX. Transabdominal pelvic ultrasound identified normal ovaries bilaterally, duplex kidneys bilaterally, and no uterus. MRI of the pelvis confirmed the duplex collecting system, normal ovaries bilaterally, and absence of Müllerian structures.

Discussion

The patient is 4 years past the onset of pubertal development. On average, menarche occurs 2 years following thelarche and correlates with a Tanner stage 3–4 breast development. Patients should be referred for evaluation of abnormal puberty (1) at age 13 if thelarche has not yet occurred, (2) 3 years post thelarche in the absence of menstruation, and (3) at age 15 years if menarche has not yet occurred in the setting of normal secondary sexual development.

In this case, the history and clinical examination demonstrate normal development of secondary sexual characteristics in the absence of a vagina, consistent with Müllerian agenesis. Pelvic ultrasound is an accurate, inexpensive, and often readily available modality to confirm the rudimentary development of the uterus.

Her 46, XX genotype eliminates the possibility of complete androgen insensitivity syndrome (CAIS), a disorder of sex development that must be considered in the differential diagnosis of vaginal agenesis [2]; see Case 3 for further discussion.

Mayer–Rokitansky–Küster–Hauser (MRKH), or congenital absence of the uterus and vagina, is prevalent in the general population affecting 1 in 4500 live female births [4]. Patients have normal ovarian tissue and function, resulting in seemingly normal pubertal development until they fail to menstruate. The paramesonephros fails to develop appropriately, leading to variable rudimentary Müllerian structures. In approximately 5 % of patients, a functional endometrium will be found within an underdeveloped uterine structure. MRKH is currently thought to result from multiple autosomal genetic and chromosomal defects [5].

MRKH must be distinguished from CAIS in which the androgen receptor is unable to recognize androgen hormones with resultant persistence of rudimentary Wolffian duct system, undescended testicular gonads, and failure to develop secondary male sexual characteristics and an absent Müllerian system. Although treatment recommendations for creating a neovagina are the same, pathogenesis and reproductive capacity are significantly different. Patients with MRKH can be reassured that ovarian tissue and function is normal and, therefore, timing and duration of hormonal changes are expected to be similar to that of the general population.

Pelvic imaging highlights the association of Müllerian anomalies with renal anomalies. Simultaneous embryologic development of the paramesonephros (Müllerian system) and metanephros (renal system) yields a 30–50 % association rate of Müllerian duct anomalies (MDA) with renal anomalies [4, 6, 7]. Vertebral and nonvertebral skeletal abnormalities are noted in approximately 7–14 % and 29–44 % of patients, respectively. Cardiac defects (16 %) and ear anomalies with and without hearing loss (up to 25 %) have been reported in several studies [8–10]. The association of cervicothoracic somite dysplasia with MDA and renal anomalies is referred to as MURCS [11].

Management

The first line treatment for creating a neovagina for girls with MRKH is vaginal self-dilation [12, 13]. The timing should be individualized to reflect the psychosocial and psychosexual maturity of the individual. Success with vaginal dilation may be improved when readiness is properly assessed prior to initiating the self-dilation process [13]. Patients who are unable to tolerate self-dilation may be a candidate for minimally invasive surgical techniques that allow for mechanical dilation, such as the modified Vecchietti or Davydov procedure [14–16]. Alternatively, graft vaginoplasty which employs skin, bowel, buccal mucosa, peritoneum, or other artificial means to create a neovagina can be used [17–20]. Concomitant psychosocial intervention may help self-image and improve sexual outcomes [21].

Patients should be reassured that there are multiple methods of creating a family. Adoption is a well-established and available process. Fertility is possible via gestational surrogacy, but may be limited by cost, cultural and ethical issues, and legal concerns. Research in the field of uterine transplant is currently in the development and exploration stages. To date, 11 uterine transplants have been performed, 7 successfully, with 1 reported live preterm birth. Further investigation will yield information regarding candidacy, safety, ethics, and reproductive outcomes [22–24].

This patient was counseled on surgical and nonsurgical options to create a neovagina by a gynecologist with experience in treating girls with vaginal agenesis. She was evaluated by a social worker with expertise in reproductive congenital anomalies for readiness using standardized and nonstandardized methods for assessing mental health; body image; commitment to treatment; and sexual maturity level including comprehension, awareness, and desire. Additionally, the logistics for privacy and personal motivation for treatment were addressed. Vaginal dilation using serial Syracuse dilators was initiated under the guidance of the gynecologist. Self-dilation instructions were provided and the method was demonstrated in the office. The patient privately employed this method for

20 minutes daily. Short-term follow-up confirmed accurate and effective technique. Interval multidisciplinary assessment of physical and psychological well-being confirmed normal neovaginal mucosa and surrounding urogenital structures and appropriate psychosocial adjustment. Fertility options were discussed but ultimately deferred.

Outcome

The patient created an 8 cm neovagina after dilating daily for 4 months. She is sexually active with a male partner. There is no dyspareunia and she reports unlimited sexual satisfaction for both herself and her partner. She has discontinued regular usage of the dilator and has been instructed to resume dilation twice weekly to maintain the neovagina in the absence of regular intercourse.

Clinical Pearls/Pitfalls

1. Vaginal agenesis should be considered in girls with amenorrhea and normal pubertal progression.
2. Müllerian agenesis is diagnosed by physical examination and confirmed with pelvic imaging.
3. Karyotyping is necessary to rule out androgen insensitivity syndromes.
4. Müllerian agenesis may be associated with renal anomalies or other congenital malformations including auditory, skeletal, cardiac, and anorectal malformations.
5. Timing and method for creating a neovagina should be individualized and based on the patient's maturity level and personal motivation. Success with self-dilation is improved with a multidisciplinary approach.
6. Girls with Müllerian agenesis are fertile despite not being unable to carry a pregnancy. Further investigation in the field of uterine transplant is warranted.

Imperforate Hymen

Case Presentation

A 12-year-old girl is referred for amenorrhea and cyclic pelvic pain for the last six months. Breast development began at age 10 years. Additional history included recent development of urinary retention and constipation. Physical examination was notable for Tanner stage 4 breasts and pubic hair development. There was no hirsutism or acne. Height was 156 cm and weight was 49 kg. The abdomen was soft, but there was a tender palpable mass above the pubic bone. There was no rebound or guarding. Examination of the external genitalia identified an imperforate hymen without any genital ambiguity. The hymen protruded with Valsalva maneuvering and with applying pressure to the suprapubic mass (Fig. 1.1a). The urethra and anus were normal.

Laboratory tests showed normal post pubertal levels of gonadotropins and normal levels of estradiol and testosterone. Transabdominal pelvic ultrasound identified a large hematometrocolpos and normal ovaries bilaterally (Fig. 1.1b).

Discussion

This patient has the classic presenting symptoms of an obstructive reproductive anomaly including normal secondary sexual characteristics, cyclic abdominal/pelvic pain, and secondary pressure symptoms. Imperforate hymen, the most common obstructive anomaly of the reproductive tract, occurs in 1 in 1000–2000 girls [25, 26]. Following several menstrual cycles, the vagina distends and cyclic pain worsens as menstrual fluid accumulates within the vaginal canal. Imperforate hymen is diagnosed on physical exam with visualization of a hymenal bulge. Pelvic imaging confirms obstruction to menstrual egress by identifying hematocolpos (see Fig. 1.1b). The differential diagnosis for amenorrhea associated with hematocolpos includes imperforate

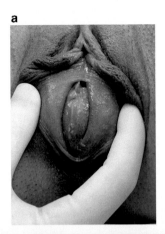

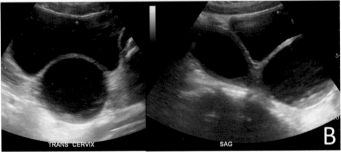

Fig. 1.1 (**a**) Imperforate hymen, (**b**) transabdominal pelvic ultrasound illustrating hematometracolpos

hymen, transverse vaginal septum, segmental vaginal agenesis, and cervical dysgenesis. Patients most often present in early adolescence; however, prenatal and neonatal diagnosis can be made when an abdominal or perineal mass consistent with a mucocolpos is noted on ultrasound or clinical examination. In neonates, a mucocolpos may be associated with other congenital anomalies, such as a cloaca malformation or persistent urogenital sinus. In the case of an isolated hymenal anomaly, surgical treatment is typically delayed until puberty unless compressive symptoms such as urinary retention, hydronephrosis, or respiratory distress develop [27, 28]. Surgical management in a symptomatic neonate should be approached by an experienced multidisciplinary surgical team in order to avoid misdiagnosis, unnecessary procedures, and potential complications [29].

The absence of a bulge upon Valsalva maneuvering or the presence of a shortened vagina without palpable cervix is concerning for a complex Müllerian duct anomaly (MDA). Pelvic MRI is needed to assess the degree and exact location of the defect within the vaginal canal to allow for adequate surgical planning [30, 31]. Transverse vaginal septum is distinguished from segmental vaginal agenesis by a thickness less than 1 cm [32]. A transverse vaginal septum can be excised and the vaginal mucosa reapproximatd with a "Z" plasty technique; however, Segmental vaginal agenesis may require preoperative dilation to reduce the distance between the upper and lower vagina or use of a graft to bridge or lengthen the vaginal canal [28]. Needle aspiration or drainage of hematocolpos should not be attempted as this can introduce bacteria into a closed and sterile environment and may lead to severe pelvic inflammatory disease or sepsis. Complications, such as endometriosis, pelvic abscess, chronic pelvic pain, or infertility associated with outflow tract obstructions can be prevented with surgical intervention to restore the conduit for menstrual egress. Referral should be made to a surgeon with specific expertise in congenital anomalies of the reproductive tract [28, 33]. Hormonal suppressive therapy should be provided if treatment delay is necessary and foley catheter insertion may be indicated to ameliorate urinary retention [34]. Laparoscopic or percutaneous drainage of the hematocolpos is a potential sterile technique which can relieve patient discomfort in patients who fail hormonal suppressive therapy and require treatment delay [35].

Management

A hymenotomy is the appropriate treatment for imperforate hymen. Foley catheter was inserted to empty the bladder and a cruciate hymenal incision allowed for decompression of the large hematocolpos with expression of copious thick brown blood (see Fig. 1.2a, b). Circumferential interrupted sutures placed to reapproximate the vaginal mucosa to the hymenal periphery was performed by a gynecologist experienced in the field of congenital reproductive anomalies (see Fig. 1.2c).

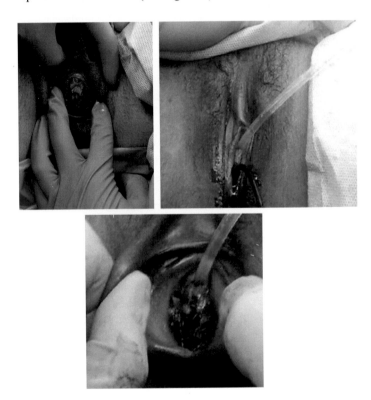

Fig. 1.2 (**a**) demarcation of the hymenal tissue outlines the cruciate incision in the hymenal tissue, (**b**) evacuation of hematocolpos, and (**c**) circumfrential interrupted sutures reapproximate the hymenal periphery to the vaginal mucosa

Outcomes

The pelvic pain resolved and the patient has regular menstrual periods. She is able to use tampons without difficulty. Postoperative dilation of the hymenal orifice is not necessary and no functional or reproductive deficits are anticipated [36].

Clinical Pearls/Pitfalls

1. Girls with normal pubertal progression, amenorrhea, and cyclic pelvic pain should be evaluated for reproductive outflow tract obstruction.
2. Imperforate hymen can be diagnosed in infancy with proper and thorough genital examination.
3. Ideal timing for hymenotomy is during early puberty, prior to menarche. Early diagnosis allows for early intervention and prevents short-term and long-term morbidity associated with outflow tract obstructions.
4. With proper surgical technique, no long-term functional or reproductive deficits are anticipated and postoperative dilation of the hymenal orifice should not be necessary

Androgen Insensitivity

Case Presentation

A 17-year-old girl is referred for primary amenorrhea. Breast and pubic hair development began at age 11 years. She is in general good health. There are no urinary complaints. She does not take any medications, vitamins, or supplements. She does not exercise regularly and she eats a healthy, balanced diet. She is not sexually active. She has no social complaints. There is a family history that is significant for two maternal aunts and a maternal cousin who did not have children.

On examination, her height is 167 cm and weight is 56 kg. Vital signs are normal. She does not have acne or hirsutism. She has sparse pubic and axillary hair and breast development is consistent with Tanner stage 5. There is a palpable mass in the left labia and in the right inguinal canal. The clitoris measures 3.5×1.2 cm on maximum stretch. The labia are normal and do not appear rugated, pigmented, or fused. There is a 2.0 cm vaginal dimple. The urethra and anus are normal.

Laboratory tests included karyotype 46, XY with positive SRY gene. Total testosterone level is 170 ng/dL, dihydrotestosterone (DHT) is 27 g/dL. Ultrasound identified absence of uterus and ovaries and confirmed right inguinal and left labial testes.

Discussion

Excess androgen hormone production in adolescent females can result in menstrual abnormalities, hirsutism, excess acne, clitormegaly, male pattern baldness, deepening of the voice and increased muscle bulk in a male distribution. The differential diagnosis associated with signs of virilization includes androgen secreting tumors, exogenous androgen exposure, late onset congenital adrenal hyperplasia, polycystic ovarian syndrome, and disorders of sexual development (DSD).

DSDs occur when the genotype of the individual is discordant with the phenotypic expression of the internal reproductive organs and/or the external genitalia of the individual [57]. 46, XX karyotype associated with late onset congenital adrenal hyperplasia is more likely to present with changes in menstrual cycle rather than primary amenorrhea. A 46, XY genotype may present with phenotypic variability ranging from genital ambiguity to normal appearing female genitalia. The DSDs associated with primary amenorrhea, genital ambiguity, and 46, XY karyotype include defects of androgen receptor function, disorders of androgen synthesis, 5 alpha reductase deficiency, and ovotesticular DSD [2, 37]. Androgen receptor impairment is differentiated from defects in testosterone synthesis or 5-alpha reductase deficiency by assessing the serum levels of testosterone and dihydrotestosterone (DHT). Androgen receptor defects can be differentiated from 5 alpha reductase deficiency because DHT production is normal in patients with androgen receptor defects and therefore the ratio of testosterone to DHT is normal.

Androgen insensitivity (AIS) is caused by a qualitative mutation in the X chromosome androgen receptor gene which makes an individual with genetic male potential resistant to the virilizing effect of testosterone and DHT. The prevalence of androgen receptor disorders is rare and approximates 1/20,000 genetic male live births [38]. These disorders are inherited as X-linked recessive and specific mutations of the receptor have been identified in families with AIS. The diagnosis of androgen receptor defect can be made by genetic sequencing. Partial androgen insensitivity (PAIS) may be due to amino acid substitutions in the hormone-binding domain of the receptor resulting in relative hormone resistance [39].

Varying degrees of androgen receptor impairment results in a relative resistance to the action of androgens. Individuals with complete androgen insensitivity (CAIS) have severe impairment of the androgen receptor function and present as normal phenotypic females with primary amenorrhea and absence of vagina and Müllerian structures (short blind ended vaginal pouch or absent vagina) with normal male testosterone levels. The Wolffian system and prostate are also absent. While both have normal breast development, these patients can be differentiated clinically from those with MRKH by the absence of axillary and pubic hair. In most cases of AIS, testes are located in the abdomen, inguinal region, or in the labia majora and testosterone levels are in the normal male range [40]. Women with PAIS have less impairment of the androgen receptor. As a result, the presenting phenotype is highly variable and the patient may present anywhere along the spectrum of a mildly virilized female to an undervirilized male with gynecomastia [39, 41]. These patients may have genital ambiguity in the setting of normal breast development and female body habitus. Pubic and axillary hair distribution varies from sparse to normal. The internal male reproductive structures may be partially or fully developed.

Optimal clinical management of individuals with DSD should include evaluation and long-term management performed at a center with an experienced multidisciplinary team including subspecialists in endocrinology, surgery, urology, gynecology, psychology, psychiatry, and genetics who are able to provide neonatal, pediatric, and adolescent care as well as transitional care into adulthood [2, 37]. Consideration should be given to the external genital appearance, genetics, internal reproductive structures, hormonal milieu, future fertility potential, and additional ethical, psychosocial, and familial issues in order to determine the gender assignment in a presenting newborn. Management for PAIS in phenotypic females is directed at preventing further manifestations of virilization at the time of puberty. Testosterone levels will decrease in response to gonadectomy. Bilateral gonadectomy is recommended to prevent malignant degeneration of cryptorchid testes. Malignancy risk varies with the DSD, location of the gonad, and patient age. Germ cell tumors and gonadoblastoma occur in about 1–4 % on undescended testes [42]. Intratubular germ cell neoplasia, a noninvasive precursor lesion has been reported in 6 % and 15 % of pediatric patients with CAIS and PAIS, respectively [43]. The lifetime risk of malignancy in patients with PAIS may be as high as 50 % and therefore gonadectomy is recommended at the time of diagnosis [37, 44, 45]. In girls with CAIS, malignancy risk is 3.6 % before age 25 years. Therefore, gonadectomy can be delayed until sexual maturation is complete so that normal pubertal growth spurt and development of secondary sexual characteristic can occur. Gonadectomy is recommended following completion of puberty as cumulative malignancy risk increases and surpasses 30 % by age 50 years [44, 46].

Gonadectomy renders the individual infertile and estrogen hormone replacement therapy is recommended to preserve bone health, minimize vasomotor symptoms, and to maintain an overall sense of well-being [33, 47, 48]. Cosmetic surgery including clito-roplasty and vaginoplasty should be determined on an individual basis and sometimes can be avoided. When surgery is indicated, emphasis should be placed on functional outcome rather than strictly on cosmetic appearance with the goal of preserving erectile function and innervation of the clitoris [2, 37]. Nonsurgical and surgical techniques for creating a neovagina are discussed above and should be deferred until the patient approaches sexual maturity. Psychological counseling for the patient and caregivers can be ben-eficial to appropriately guide the child as she approaches different psychosocial milestones [47–49]. The data regarding psychologic outcomes in patients with DSD is often reported as a collective group rather than a single diagnosis given the rarity of these condi-tions and further studies are needed to clarify disease-specific psy-chological implications. Despite a lack of data specific to AIS, expert opinion and cumulative data support the assistance of a therapist experienced with DSD to help guide the patient and fam-ily through cognitively appropriate disclosure of the diagnosis and to aid with gender identity [48]. This is a critical component of patient care, as DSD patients have been shown to have high rates of suicidal thoughts and anxiety compared to controls [50]. Teens with DSD have fewer close friendships and love experiences com-pared to their peers, and as adults 46XY women demonstrate lower femininity scores [51]. In a study of patients with XY DSD, patients reported higher fear of sexual contact, decreased sexual desire, increased issues with arousal, increased sexual pain, and higher rates of dissatisfaction with their overall sex life compared to con-trols [52].

Androgen insensitivity syndromes are generally considered incompatible with fertility. Due to the SRY gene, the Müllerian structures regress. In patients with CAIS, the Wolffiann system is also underdeveloped. Changes in gonadal histology, including loss of germ cells and tubular atrophy take place in early childhood [43]. While successful uterine transplantation and pregnancy fol-lowing IVF have recently been reported, all patients had a 46XX karyotype and uterine infertility due to agenesis or hysterectomy

[22, 23]. The role of uterine transplantation in patients with DSD has not yet been explored, but a review of patients who applied for the uterine transplant project at Akdeniz University Hospital demonstrated that 8.4 % of applicants had CAIS [53]. The feasibility of uterine transplant in DSD patients is unknown given differences in anatomy, requirements for donor oocytes and hormonal support and ethical consideration.

Patients with PAIS have variable development of the Wolffian system and prostate. Literature review demonstrates case reports of male patients with mild PAIS who have been able to preserve fertility. Clinically, these patients present as undervirilized males with gynecomastia and have low ejaculation and/or semen volumes [39] or conceive spontaneously [54]. Assisted reproductive technologies, such as testicular extraction of sperm with intracytoplasmic sperm injection may be necessary to overcome these obstacles [55, 56].

Optimal care of the individual with a DSD requires the attention from a multidisciplinary team of specialists. Ideally, a comprehensive team is comprised of specialists in the fields of endocrinology, urology, gynecology, genetics, and mental health professionals who appreciate the unique issues pertaining to caring for these individuals, including issues related to sex assignment, gender identity, sexual orientation, sexual functioning, pubertal development, fertility potential, body image, and overall psychosocial well-being of the patients and their caregivers.

Management

In this case, psychosocial assessment confirmed a female sexual identity and an adequate understanding of her diagnosis. The patient underwent a bilateral gonadectomy and a nerve sparing clitoroplasty. She was started on an estradiol patch for hormone replacement therapy to preserve bone health and overall sense of well-being. Progesterone was not indicated due to the lack of Müllerian structures and menses was not anticipated. Postoperatively, she was instructed to apply moderate pressure to the vaginal mucosa with a dilator for 20 min each day in order to create a neovagina using native mucosa and serial dilations. Psychosocial assessment and intervention with a social worker who is knowledgeable about the issues pertaining to individuals with DSDs was maintained throughout her care.

Outcomes

She is tolerating the hormone replacement therapy well. She is psychosocially well adjusted. There are no urinary complaints and clitoral sensation is uncompromised. A neovagina was successfully created with progressive perineal self-dilation. She is sexually active with one male partner without difficulty. Usage of the dilator has been discontinued. She continues to follow up with the multidisciplinary group of physicians and a social worker who specializes caring for patients with DSD.

Clinical Pearls and Pitfalls

1. Karyotyping and genetic testing are useful tools in evaluating patients with primary amenorrhea and genital ambiguity.
2. DSDs occur when the genotype and the phenotype of an individual are discordant.
3. Individuals with DSD and a female sex assignment often experience primary amenorrhea.
4. Gonadectomy is recommended for patients with androgen insensitivity syndromes to prevent malignant transformation of the testes and to prevent virilization effects for patients with incomplete androgen receptor defects who have a female sexual identity. Gonadectomy is recommended at the time of diagnosis in patients with PAIS, but can be delayed until puberty is complete in patients with CAIS.
5. Hormone replacement therapy is necessary following gonadectomy.

6. Cosmetic genital surgery including clitoroplasty, labiaplasty, and vaginoplasty are not mandatory and should be based on individual preference.
7. Optimal care of the individual with a DSD requires a multidisciplinary approach with a team of specialists which should include an endocrinologist, gynecologist, urologist, geneticist, and mental health professional who are experienced in caring for patients with DSDs.

Summary

These cases illustrate the importance of considering congenital disorders for girls with primary amenorrhea. The diagnostic approach to various forms of structural defects emphasizes the importance of physical examination in the evaluation of girls with primary amenorrhea. Pelvic imaging is necessary to guide surgical intervention and chromosomal assessment is imperative for appropriate diagnosis and fertility counseling.

References

1. Practice Committee of the American Society for Reproductive Medicine. Current evaluation of amenorrhea. Fertil Steril. 2008;90(S3):S219–25.
2. Ahmed SF, Achermann JC, Arlt W, et al. UK guidance on the initial evaluation of an infant or an adolescent with a suspected disorder of sex development. Clin Endocrinol (Oxf). 2011;75(1):12–26.
3. Emans SJ. Education of the child and adolescent. In: Emans SJ, Laufer MR, Goldstein DP, editors. Pediatric and adolescent gynecology. 5th ed. Philadelphia: Lippincott Williams & Wilkins; 2005. p. 487–90.
4. Oppelt PG, Lermann J, Strick R, Dittrich R, Strissel P, Rettig I, Schulze C, Renner SP, Beckmann MW, Brucker S, Rall K, Mueller A. Malformations in a cohort of 284 women with Mayer-Rokitansky-Küster-Hauser syndrome (MRKH). Reprod Biol Endocrinol. 2012;10(1):57.
5. Patnaik SS, Brazile B, Dandolu V, Ryan PL, Liao J. Mayer-Rokitansky-Küster-Hauser (MRKH) syndrome: A historical perspective. Gene. 2015;555(1):33–40.

6. Price TM, Bates GW. Adolescent amenorrhea (Chapter 13). In: Koehler Carpenter SE, Rock JA, editors. Pediatric and adolescent gynecology. 2nd ed. Philadelphia: Lippincott Williams & Wilkins; 2000. p. 183–5.

7. Sajjad Y. Development of the genital ducts and external genitalia in the early human embryo. J Obstet Gynaecol Res. 2010;36(5):929–37.

8. Kimberley N, Hutson JM, Southwell BR, Grover SR. Vaginal agenesis, the hymen, and associated anomalies. J Pediatr Adolesc Gynecol. 2012;25(1): 54–8.

9. Li S, Qayyum A, Coakley FV, Hricak H. Association of renal agenesis and Mullerian duct anomalies. J Comput Assist Tomogr. 2000;24(6):829–34.

10. Pittock ST, Babovic-Vuksanovic D, Lteir A. Mayer-Rokitansky-Küster-Hauser anomaly and its associated malformations. Am J Med Genet A. 2005;135(3):314–6.

11. Duncan PA, Shapiro L, Stangel JJ, Klein RM, Addonizio J. The MURCS Association: Mullerian duct aplasia, renal aplasia, and cervicothoracic somite dysplasia. J Pediatr. 1979;95(3):399–402.

12. ACOG. Müllerian agenesis: diagnosis, management, and treatment. Committee Opinion No. 562. Obstet Gynecol. 2013;121:1134–7.

13. Edmonds DK. Management of vaginal agenesis. Curr Opin Obstet Gynecol. 2013;25(5):382–7.

14. Brucker SY, Gegusch M, Zubke W, Rall K, Gauwerky JF, Wallwiener D. Neovagina creation in vaginal agenesis: development of a new laparoscopic Vecchietti-based procedure and optimized instruments in a prospective comparative interventional study in 101 patients. Fertil Steril. 2008;90(5):1940–52.

15. Fedele L, Bianchi S, Zanconato G, Raffaelli R. Laparoscopic creation of a neovagina in patients with Rokitansky syndrome: analysis of 52 cases. Fertil Steril. 2000;74(2):384–9.

16. Fedele L, Frontino G, Restelli E, Ciappina N, Motta F, Bianchi S. Creation of a neovagina by Davydov's laparoscopic modified technique in patients with Rokitansky syndrome. Am J Obstet Gynecol. 2010;202(1):33.

17. Darai E, Toullalan O, Besse O, PoritonL DP. Anatomic and functional results of laparoscopic-perineal. Hum Reprod. 2003;18:2454–9.

18. Dargent D, Marchiole P, Giannesi A, Benchaib M, Chevret-Measson M, Mathevet P. Laparoscopic Davydov or laparoscopic transposition of the peritoneum colpopoiesis described by Davydov for the treatment of genital vaginal agenesis: the technique and its evolution. Gynecol Obstet Fertil. 2004;32:1023–30.

19. Grimsby GM, Baker LA. The use of autologous buccal mucosa grafts in vaginal reconstruction. Curr Urol Rep. 2014;15(8):428.

20. Roberts CP, Haber MJ, Rock JA. Vaginal creation for Müllerian agenesis. Am J Obstet Gynecol. 2001;185(6):1349–52.

21. Bean EJ, Mazur T, Robinson AD. Mayer-Rokitansky-Küster-Hauser syndrome: sexuality, psychological effects, and quality of life. J Pediatr Adolesc Gynecol. 2009;22(6):339–46.

22. Brännström M, Johannesson L, Bokström H, Kvarnström N, Mölne J, Dahm-Kähler P, Enskog A, Milenkovic M, Ekberg J, Diaz-Garcia C, Gäbel M, Hanafy A, Hagberg H, Olausson M, Nilsson L. Livebirth after uterus transplantation. Lancet. 2014;pii:S0140-6736(14)61729-1.

23. Brännström M, Johannesson L, Dahm-Kähler P, Enskog A, Mölne J, Kvarnström N, Diaz-Garcia C, Hanafy A, Lundmark C, Marcickiewicz J, Gäbel M, Groth K, Akouri R, Eklind S, Holgersson J, Tzakis A, Olausson M. First clinical uterus transplantation trial: a six-month report. Fertil Steril. 2014;101(5):1228–36. doi:10.1016/j.fertnstert.2014.02.024.

24. Olausson M, Johannesson L, Brattgård D, Diaz-Garcia C, Lundmark C, Groth K, Marcickiewizc J, Enskog A, Akouri R, Tzakis A, Rogiers X, Janson PO, Brännström M. Ethics of uterus transplantation with live donors. Fertil Steril. 2014;120(1):40–3.

25. Breech LL, Laufer MR. Mullerian anomalies. Obstet Gynecol Clin North Am. 2009;36:47–68.

26. Dietrich JE, Millar DM, Quint EH. Obstructive reproductive tract anomalies. J Pediatr Adolesc Gynecol. 2014;27(6):396–402.

27. Ameh EA, Mshelbwala PM, Ameh N. Congenital vaginal obstruction in neonates and infants: recognition and management. J Pediatr Adolesc Gynecol. 2011;2011(2):74–8.

28. Miller RJ, Breech LL. Surgical correction of vaginal anomalies. Clin Obstet Gynecol. 2008;51(2):223–36.

29. Nazir Z, Rizvi RM, Qureshi RN, Khan ZS, Khan Z. Congenital vaginal obstructions: varied presentation and outcome. Pediatr Surg Int. 2006; 22(9):749–53.

30. Church DG, Vancil JM, Vasanawala SS. Magnetic resonance imaging for uterine and vaginal anomalies. Curr Opin Obstet Gynecol. 2009;21(5): 379–89.

31. Humphries PD, Simpson JC, Creighton SM, Hall-Craggs MA. MRI in the assessment of congenital vaginal anomalies. Clin Radiol. 2008;63(4): 442–8.

32. Wierrani F, Bodner K, Spängler B, Grünberger W. "Z"-plasty of the transverse vaginal septum using Garcia's procedure and the Grünberger modification. Fertil Steril. 2003;79(3):608–12.

33. Bertelloni S, Dati E, Baroncelli GI. Disorders of sex development: hormonal management in adolescence. Gynecol Endocrinol. 2008;24(6):339–46. doi:10.1080/09513590802055708.

34. Christodoulidou M, Kaba R, Oates J, Wemyss-Holden GD. Acute urinary retention in an adolescent girl and important learning points. BMJ Case Rep. 2013;pii: bcr2013010361. doi: 10.1136/bcr-2013-010361.

35. Dennie J, Pillay S, Watson D, Grover S. Laparoscopic drainage of hematocolpos: a new treatment option for the acute management of a transverse vaginal septum. Fertil Steril. 2010;94(5):1853–7.

36. Joki-Erkkilä MM, Heinonen PK. Presenting and long-term clinical implications and fecundity in females with obstructing vaginal malformations. J Pediatr Adolesc Gynecol. 2003;16(5):307–12.

37. Lee PA, Houk CP, Ahmed SF, Hughes IA, International Consensus Conference on Intersex organized by the Lawson Wilkins Pediatric Endocrine Society and the European Society for Paediatric Endocrinology. Consensus statement on management of intersex disorders. International Consensus Conference on Intersex. Pediatrics. 2008;118(2):e488–500.
38. Bangsbøll S, Qvist I, Lebech PE, Lewinsky M. Testicular feminization syndrome and associated gonadal tumors in Denmark. Acta Obstet Gynecol Scand. 1992;71(1):63–6.
39. Grino PB, Griffin JE, Cushard Jr WG, Wilson JD. A mutation of the androgen receptor associated with partial androgen resistance, familial gynecomastia, and fertility. J Clin Endocrinol Metab. 1988;66(4):754–61.
40. Quigley CA, De Bellis A, Marschke KB, El-Awady MK, Wilson EM, French FS. Androgen receptor defects: historical, clinical, and molecular perspectives. Endocr Rev. 1995;16(3):271–321.
41. Brinkmann AO. Molecular basis of androgen insensitivity. Mol Cell Endocrinol. 2001;179(1–2):105–9.
42. Wood HM, Elder JS. Cryptorchidism and testicular cancer: separating fact from fiction. J Urol. 2009;181:452–61.
43. Kaprova-Pleskacova J, Stoop H, Brüggenwirth H, Cools M, Wolffenbuttel KP, Drop SL, Snajderova M, Lebl J, Oosterhuis JW, Looijenga LH. Complete androgen insensitivity syndrome: factors influencing gonadal histology including germ cell pathology. Mod Pathol. 2014;27(5):721–30. doi:10.1038/modpathol.2013.193.
44. Levin HS. Tumors of the testis in intersex syndromes. Urol Clin North Am. 2000;27(3):543–51.
45. Ramani P, Yeung CK, Habeebu SS. Testicular intratubular germ cell neoplasia in children and adolescents with intersex. Am J Surg Pathol. 1993; 17(11):1124–33.
46. Manuel M, Katayama KP, Jones HW. The age of occurrence of gonadal tumors in intersex patients with Y chromosome. Am J Obstet Gynecol. 1976;124:293–300.
47. Jorgensen PB, Kjartansdóttir KR, Fedder J. Care of women with XY karyotype: a clinical practice guideline. Fertil Steril. 2010;94(1):105–13. doi:10.1016/j.fertnstert.2009.02.087.
48. Oakes MB, Eyvazzadeh AD, Quint E, Smith YR. Complete androgen insensitivity syndrome - A review. J Pediatr Adolesc Gynecol. 2008; 21(6):305–10.
49. Slijper FM, Frets PG, Boehmer AL, Drop SL, Niermeijer MF. Androgen insensitivity syndrome (AIS): emotional reactions of parents and adult patients to the clinical diagnosis of AIS and its confirmation by androgen receptor gene mutation analysis. Horm Res. 2000;53(1):9–15.
50. Johannsen TH, Ripa CP, Mortensen EL, Main KM. Quality of life in 70 women with disorders of sex development. Eur J Endocrinol. 2006; 155:877–85.
51. Jürgensen M, Kleinemeier E, Lux A, Steensma TD, Cohen-Kettenis PT, Hiort O, Thyen U, Köhler B, Network Working Group DSD. Psychosexual

development in adolescents and adults with disorders of sex development--results from the German Clinical Evaluation Study. J Sex Med. 2013;10(11):2703–14. doi:10.1111/j.1743-6109.2012.02751.x.

52. Köhler B, Kleinemeier E, Lux A, Hiort O, Grüters A, Thyen U, Network Working Group DSD. Satisfaction with genital surgery and sexual life of adults with XY disorders of sex development: results from the German clinical evaluation study. J Clin Endocrinol Metab. 2012;97(2):577–88. doi:10.1210/jc.2011-1441.

53. Erman Akar M, Ozekinci M, Alper O, Demir D, Cevikol C, Meric Bilekdemir A, Daloglu A, Ongut G, Senol Y, Ozdem S, Uzun G, Luleci G, Suleymanlar G. Assessment of women who applied for the uterine transplant project as potential candidates for uterus transplantation. J Obstet Gynaecol Res. 2015;41(1):12–6.

54. Giwercman A, Kledal T, Schwartz M, Giwercman YL, Leffers H, Zazzi H, Wedell A, Skakkebaek NE. Preserved male fertility despite decreased androgen sensitivity caused by a mutation in the ligand-binding domain of the androgen receptor gene. J Clin Endocrinol Metab. 2000;85(6):2253–9.

55. Massin N, Bry H, Vija L, Maione L, Constancis E, Haddad B, Morel Y, Claessens F, Young J. Healthy birth after testicular extraction of sperm and ICSI from an azoospermic man with mild androgen insensitivity syndrome caused by an androgen receptor partial loss-of-function mutation. Clin Endocrinol(Oxf).2012;77(4):593–8.doi:10.1111/j.1365-2265.2012.04402.x.

56. Tordjman KM, Yaron M, Berkovitz A, Botchan A, Sultan C, Lumbroso S. Fertility after high-dose testosterone and intracytoplasmic sperm injection in a patient with androgen insensitivity syndrome with a previously unreported androgen receptor mutation. Andrologia. 2013;46(6):703–6.

57. Evans TN, Poland ML, Boving RL. Vaginal malformations. Am J Obstet Gynecol. 1981;141(8):910–20.

Chapter 2
Precocious Puberty

Jason Klein and Patricia M. Vuguin

Abbreviations

BMI	Body mass index
CPP	Central precocious puberty
GDPP	Gonadotropin-dependent precocious puberty
GIPP	Gonadotropin-independent precocious puberty
GnRH	Gonadotropin-releasing hormone
MAS	McCune–Albright syndrome
PP	Precocious puberty
PPP	Peripheral precocious puberty
TBI	Traumatic brain injury

J. Klein, M.D. (✉)
Division of Pediatric Endocrinology, Cohen Children's Medical
Center of NY, 1991 Marcus Avenue, Suite M100,
Lake Success, NY 11042, USA

Hofstra Northwell School of Medicine, Hempstead,
NY 11549, USA
e-mail: jklein3@nshs.edu

P.M. Vuguin, M.Sc., M.D.
Hofstra Northwell School of Medicine, Hempstead,
NY 11549, USA
e-mail: pvuguin@nshs.edu

© Springer International Publishing Switzerland 2016
H.L. Appelbaum (ed.), *Abnormal Female Puberty*,
DOI 10.1007/978-3-319-27225-2_2

Introduction

Puberty is defined as the transition from sexual immaturity to sexual maturity. The two main physiological events that occur during puberty include the activation of the gonads by the pituitary hormones also known as "gonadarche" and the production of androgens by the adrenal cortex also known as "adrenarche."

The normal onset, progression, tempo, and completion of female puberty require a complex series of genetic and hormonal interactions, working together in biological and psychological concert. This is a gradual process with hypothalamic GnRH neurons, called the "gonadostat," triggering a hormonal cascade and eventually resulting in the physical changes associated with puberty. The initial clinical sign of female puberty is breast development, or thelarche, which normally occurs between the ages of 8 and 13 years. Early, or precocious, puberty (PP) in females is defined as the appearance of thelarche at an age 2.5–3 standard deviations (SD) below the mean age of onset of puberty [1]. In the United States, the traditional definition of PP—thelarche before the age of 8 years old—is still an ongoing debate. It has been recommended that girls who develop signs of puberty between 7 and 8 years of age, the evaluation will depend on the degree, tempo of maturation, and family history [2]. Girls are nearly 12 times more likely to develop precocious puberty when compared with their male counterparts [3].

The causes of precocious puberty are expansive, ranging from variants of normal development to certain genetic syndromes to pathologic conditions with and/or without significant risks of morbidity and mortality. Evaluation involves a complete and thorough history and physical examination, detailing the signs of development, including when these signs began, the timing and progression of these signs, and associated changes in growth. Girls with true precocious puberty, in addition to physical findings of thelarche and pubarche (pubic hair), have early growth acceleration, premature bone maturation, and initially become taller than their peers, but, untreated, ultimately achieve shorter than predicted final adult heights due to premature epiphyseal fusion.

Laboratory analysis of gonadotropins and estradiol will help confirm the presence of true precocious puberty, as well as localize the source of hormone production. Two classifications of precocious puberty include central precocious puberty (CPP), under the influence of pituitary control, or peripheral precocious puberty (PPP), which is secondary to estrogen production outside the influence of pituitary control. Subsequent targeted imaging and/or more specific testing will lead the clinician to a particular etiology. This chapter will provide a case-based review of several causes of precocious puberty in girls as well as discuss diagnostic and treatment modalities.

Brain Tumor

Case Presentation

A 3.5-year-old girl is referred for evaluation of pubic hair and breast development. The pubic hair was first noted approximately 6 months ago. At a recent well-child physical approximately 1 month ago, she was noted to have developed breast tissue, and she was referred for an endocrinological evaluation. While waiting for this endocrine appointment, there were two times that the parents noted dried blood in her pull-up diaper. She has been otherwise healthy with no other medical problems. She is developmentally appropriate and in pre-kindergarten classes. There is no significant family history. Mother's height is 62 in. and father's height is 66 in. Family denies any environmental exposures of exogenous hormones.

On examination, her height is 105 cm (41 in.) at the 75th percentile and weight was 17 kg (38 lb) at the 72nd percentile; BMI was 15.9 kg/m^2 at the 68th percentile. Review of her prior growth curves shows that she was measured at the 25th percentile for height at age 3 years. Her blood pressure is normal. She has no acne, hirsutism, or cutaneous findings. Pubertal status is Tanner stage 3–4 for breasts with estrogenization of the aerolae. Pubic hair is Tanner 3. There is scant axillary hair. The vaginal mucosa appears slightly pink with minimal discharge. There is no clitoral enlargement.

Early morning laboratory testing shows elevated gonadotropins (FSH 6.2 mIU/mL and LH 3.1 mIU/mL) and elevated estradiol of 27 pg/mL (normal range for prepubertal girls 5–20 pg/mL). 17-Hydroxyprogesterone is normal. Bone age X-ray is performed and read as advanced with a skeletal age of 6 years. MRI of the head/pituitary with and without contrast is performed, revealing a well-defined pedunculated hypothalamic mass, measuring 3.4×2.6 cm.

Discussion

This girl has developed glandular breast tissue (thelarche) prior to the age of 8 years in context of pubic hair growth (pubarche) and growth acceleration, consistent with PP. While most pediatric endocrinologists agree with 8 years as the lower limit of the normal onset of puberty in females, studies have shown that there may be racial differences as well as a general drift towards earlier onset puberty, with African American girls as young as 6 years and Hispanic and Caucasian girls as young as 7 years going into puberty without impacting growth potential [4, 5]. In addition, the increasing obesity epidemic in the pediatric population may play a role in this possible decreasing age of pubertal onset [6, 7]. Certain environmental exposures, including contact with exogenous hormones, have been implicated in cases of precocious puberty.

When examining children with concern for precocious puberty, it is important to consider normal variants of pubertal development as a possible alternate diagnosis. Premature thelarche, or isolated breast development without other signs of puberty, is a common and benign condition in girls younger than 3 years old and is often mistaken for precocious puberty. These children do not have pubarche nor growth acceleration or advanced bone ages [3, 7]. FSH levels tend to be elevated, though LH remains in the prepubertal range. Estradiol may intermittently rise into the early pubertal range, though this is not sustained. The breast tissue in these girls tends to regress or even completely resolve, and they will go on to have a normally timed onset of puberty and menarche. Estrogenization of the aerolae, which appears as darkening and enlargement, may be present in these cases, though typically not as marked as in true PP. Premature adrenarche, which may present as apocrine body odor, acne, or axillary and/or pubic hair development before age 8 years, is due to early activation of adrenal androgen production. Children with PA have been shown to exhibit higher early morning serum levels of dehydroepiandrosterone (DHEA), dehydroepiandrosterone sulfate (DHEA-S), androstenedione, testosterone, pregnenolone, and 17-OH-progesterone. The serum concentration of DHEA-S is the best marker for the presence of adrenarche (level greater than 40 μg/dL). The androgen levels in the above case are consistent with early Tanner II-III [8–10]. Levels of DHEAS >750 μg/dL or testosterone >150 ng/dL should prompt evaluation for androgen-producing tumor. Patients with benign premature adrenarche do not have thelarche, growth acceleration, or advanced bone ages. It is important to rule out non-classic congenital adrenal hyperplasia in these patients by way of an early morning (~8 AM) 17-OH-progesterone level. Girls with CAH will first show signs of early adrenarche, though this can stimulate CPP [3, 7]. Of note, girls who have premature adrenarche in youth may be at risk for developing insulin resistance and polycystic ovarian syndrome (PCOS) in adolescence or later, with some studies citing up to a 15–20 % risk [11–14].

In this case, the patient's labs show elevated gonadotropins and estradiol levels, consistent with central, or gonadotropin-dependent, precocious puberty (GDPP). The most common cause of GDPP in females, in approximately 75 % of cases, is idiopathic [3, 7]. Out of identifiable causes, CNS/hypothalamic tumors are the most common etiology, making up 5–10 % of GDPP cases in female patients [15].

Hypothalamic hamartomas are congenital, non-neoplastic, heterotopic masses of neurons, glia, and fiber bundles that arise from the floor of the third ventricle, tuber cinereum, or mammillary bodies. The prevalence of these CNS masses is thought to be 1–2 per 100,000 and can present with gelastic seizures or other epilepsy, cognitive impairment, psychiatric disorders, or other developmental problems [16, 17]. GDPP secondary to hypothalamic hamartoma is common in younger children, being described in as young as infancy and typically occurring before age 4 years. The method by which the hypothalamic hamartoma results in GDPP is thought to be due to tumor-related production of pulsatile LH-releasing hormone, thereby overcoming the normal hypothalamic pubertal inhibition [18].

While overall more common in boys with GDPP than girls with GDPP, hypothalamic hamartomas are the classic CNS tumor associated with sexual precocity. Other CNS lesions that may result in CPP include astrocytoma [19], ependymoma, pineal tumors, and optic and hypothalamic gliomas. Patients with neurofibromatosis type 1 (von Recklinghausen disease) in particular may have precocious puberty in association with optic gliomas [20], though precocity may still appear in their absence [21].

The decision to order imaging studies is based on the clinical impression and results of the initial laboratory evaluation. Any physical of laboratory findings suggesting autonomously functioning ovarian cysts or ovarian tumors are indications to obtain a pelvic ultrasound. Pelvic ultrasonography is not indicated as part of the workup in cases of GDPP as there is no focal ovarian pathology. Pelvic ultrasound could be used to monitor pubertal progress in girls; with uterine volume changes above 2 mL suggest progressive puberty. Should a transabdominal pelvic ultrasound be performed in a patient with GDPP, one may simply see an increase in size of the uterus and ovaries similar to that of a pubertal female, possibly with multicystic ovaries; these ovarian changes may not regress following GnRH analogue treatment, though this does not appear to have any clinical implications [22].

Rarely, severe undiagnosed hypothyroidism may result in precocious puberty; the mechanism is not completely understood though thought to be due to increased TRH activation of gonadotropes. Treatment with levothyroxine will reverse the precocious puberty [23, 24].

Management

The primary physical result of untreated precocious puberty is short final adult height due to premature fusion of the epiphyseal growth plates under the influence of excess estrogen production. In addition to the physical, there may be cases in which the final adult height is not impacted, but psychological or psychosocial aspects of early puberty may be worrisome to the patient and/or the family. Precocity of secondary sexual characteristics has been linked to aggression, delinquency, negative self-image, and an increased risk of possible sexual exploitation/abuse [25–27]. Should children be seen by their parents or caregivers as too immature to handle physical changes associated with puberty, treatment may be indicated. In these cases of idiopathic GDPP, treatment to suppress pituitary gonadotropins using GnRH agonists, as detailed below, would be indicated.

FSH and LH rise in puberty due to the pulsatile release of GnRH from the hypothalamus [4, 5]. GnRH agonists, such as the monthly or quarterly leuprolide acetate depot IM injection or yearly histrelin subdermal implantation, will introduce a constant, non-pulsatile GnRH milieu, effectively desensitizing and decreasing gonadotropin release. The choice of formulation depends on family, the clinician, and the insurance preference. These formulations have not been directly compared to each other in randomized trials, but appear to have a similar effect in suppressing the axis. Response is judged on subsequent physical examination, during which signs of puberty should be noted to have stopped progressing and then to regress over the first 6 months of treatment. Growth velocity should return to a typical prepubertal rate. Gonadotropin and estradiol levels should decrease to prepubertal levels within a month following treatment. Labs should be routinely monitored during treatment, as should the bone age. Patients who do not have very advanced bone ages prior to treatment tend to have better results with respect to gaining back their height potential [3, 28]. Discontinuation of therapy should be based on the patient's age, growth velocity, bone age, height prediction, and psychosocial readiness. Treatment with GnRH agonists appears to have no significant long-term effects on the pituitary–gonadal axis. Bone density may decrease during prolonged therapy, but is regained after treatment, therefore monitoring of bone density is not required.

Treatment of hypothalamic hamartoma is directed towards its removal, especially in those who have frequent seizures as a result of the mass. Over the past 2 decades, newer advances in surgical approach, including microsurgery, gamma knife surgery and stereotactic radiosurgery, and radiofrequency ablation, have allowed neurosurgeons to treat patients with minimal complications [29].

Outcome

The patient underwent placement of a histrelin implant, which halted further progression of puberty. Repeat labs ~3 months after implant showed prepubertal levels of FSH and estradiol; LH remained in the early pubertal range. She was referred to neurosurgery for her hypothalamic hamartoma, and the family elected to observe the mass with repeat MRI in 6 months. During the interval, though, the patient developed a seizure and the mass ultimately required resection. No further seizure activity occurred and her examination 1 year after treatment was significantly improved with near regression of all pubertal signs.

Clinical Pearls/Pitfalls

1. Central or gonadotropin-dependent precocious puberty is the most common cause of precocious puberty in females.
2. The first sign of puberty in females is thelarche in context of growth acceleration, advanced bone age, and possibly pubarche.
3. Laboratory testing will reveal elevated gonadotropins and estradiol; MRI of the brain is the diagnostic imaging of choice.
4. Following appropriate evaluation, most patients are found to have idiopathic GDPP.
5. CNS tumors, specifically hypothalamic hamartomas, are the leading identifiable cause of female CPP in young patients.
6. Treatment of CPP may involve GnRH agonist to suppress further gonadotropin release.

Ovarian Cyst

Case Presentation

A 4.5-year-old girl is referred for evaluation of breast development and vaginal discharge. Her family states that she has been noted to have progressive breast enlargement over the preceding

6 months. This was first noted when the patient's mother was holding her and felt "a lump" on her chest. This concern was brought to the attention of the pediatrician, who reassured the family. Over the past 2 weeks, she has been noted to have some whitish appearing vaginal discharge. There has not been any pubic or axillary hair growth nor any acne or adult body odors. Her family states that there was one time, approximately 3 weeks ago, that they noted some dried blood in her underwear. Her general health has been otherwise good, and she has no other medical issues. Family denies any environmental exposure. Review of her growth curves shows increased height percentile since last year, from the 25th percentile to the now ~50th.

On examination, her height is 105 cm (41 in.) at the 56th percentile and weight is 16.5 kg (36.5 lb) at the 43rd percentile; BMI is 14.9 kg/m^2 at the 41st percentile. Her blood pressure is normal. She has no acne, hirsutism, or cutaneous findings. Pubertal status is Tanner stage 2 for breasts with estrogenization of aerolae. Pubic hair is Tanner 1. The vaginal mucosa appears slightly pink with mild discharge. There is no clitoral enlargement.

Laboratory testing included gonadotropins and estradiol. Follicle-stimulating hormone (FSH) is 0.085 mIU/mL and luteinizing hormone (LH) is 0.01 mIU/mL, both low and in the prepubertal range. Estradiol is elevated at 270 pg/mL. Bone age X-ray is performed and read as consistent with the patient's chronologic age. Transabdominal pelvic ultrasound identifies a left ovarian simple cyst, measuring 3.8 cm. Endometrial thickness is 2 mm and within normal limits for age.

Discussion

Similar to the first case, this patient also has precocious puberty, evidenced by the presence of thelarche prior to the age of 8 years in association with growth acceleration. In this situation, though, while the estradiol is extremely elevated, the gonadotropins are suppressed. This is consistent with peripheral, or gonadotropin-independent, precocious puberty. GIPP in females is secondary to autonomous secretion of ovarian estrogens (via cyst, tumor, or non-gonadotropin stimulation), adrenal neoplasm, or exogenous exposures to estrogens [5].

The most common cause of GIPP is autonomously functioning ovarian follicular cysts [30]. GIPP should be strongly considered in the differential diagnosis where thelarche is the predominant or initial sign of pubertal development (as opposed to pubarche). As detailed earlier, it is important to distinguish benign premature thelarche, the presence of breast tissue without other signs of puberty, from PP; girls with benign premature thelarche do not have growth acceleration or an advanced bone age.

If a diagnosis of precocious puberty is made in context of an autonomously functioning ovarian cyst, the patient should be evaluated for possible McCune–Albright syndrome (MAS). MAS is a genetic condition in which a somatic mutation in the GNAS1 gene results in constitutively activating the $G_s\alpha$ protein present in many tissues. In addition to GIPP, the classic findings of the syndrome include large café-au-lait macules with irregular borders (referred to as "coast of Maine" in appearance) and polyosteotic fibrous dysplasia, a slowly progressive bone disorder [5]. Hyperfunctioning autonomous endocrinopathies in MAS are typically associated with the ovary, though due to the presence of the $G_s\alpha$ protein in the receptor for other pituitary hormones, patients with MAS may also develop hyperthyroidism, Cushing syndrome, gigantism/acromegaly, or hyperparathyroidism. Diagnostic workup for these patients involves skeletal X-rays to look for the bony findings of MAS, as well as endocrine investigation for these other associated conditions.

Ovarian tumors are rare in the prepubertal period and usually present with abdominal pain or distention, though they may present with signs of virilization or early puberty. While adult ovarian tumors tend to arise from the ovarian epithelium, pediatric tumors usually originate from germ cells or sex cord-stromal cells [31]. The most common of these rare tumors is the granulosa cell tumor, followed by the theca cell tumor and sex cord-stromal cell tumors. Estrogen may be produced by the tumor and result in signs of precocious puberty. Tumor markers, anti-Mullerian hormone (AMH) and inhibin, can be used for screening or during recovery [32]. Sex cord-stromal cell tumors may result in elevated testosterone levels and should be examined in context of possible Peutz–Jeghers syndrome, a condition characterized by mucocutaneous hyperpigmentation, gastrointestinal hamartomatous polyposis, and an increased risk of malignancy due to a mutation in serine/threonine kinase 11 (STK11), a tumor-suppressing gene [33]. Surgical resection is the treatment of choice for ovarian tumors and in young girls prognosis tends to be favorable.

Transabdominal pelvic ultrasound in a patient with GIPP may identify a large tumor or one or more cysts of the ovary. Small, unilocular ovarian cysts of less than 1 cm in diameter in prepubertal girls are clinically insignificant, while ovarian cysts associated with GIPP are generally larger than 2 cm in diameter [34].

Management

Most autonomously functioning ovarian cysts will spontaneously involute, thereby removing the estrogen production and causing the precocious puberty to regress. Surgical excision of the cyst is reserved for refractory cases, complex ovarian masses, or large cysts where there is a risk for ovarian torsion [35]. Those patients who do not meet criteria for surgery can be clinically monitored with examination and repeat labs and ultrasound every 6 weeks.

In contrast, patients with MAS have a somatic (postzygotic) mutation of the alpha subunit of the G3 protein that leads to continued stimulation of endocrine function. Thus, for those patients who have progressive GIPP, simple observation may not be appropriate as functional ovarian cysts may not spontaneously involute, and new cysts will invariably develop. Medical therapy with aromatase inhibitors such as Letrozole, which block the production of estrogens, and estrogen-receptor modulators such as Tamoxifen have been attempted with success as adjuvant therapy with surgical resection of large cysts, though with limited patient data and no long-term outcome studies [36, 37].

Outcome

The patient was initially observed clinically over the next month, during which time her breast development began to regress. Repeat ultrasound showed a similarly sized cyst, though with newly noted possible septations. Due to change in appearance, she was referred to pediatric surgery for consultation, who recommended continued observation. Three months later, the cyst had nearly completely involuted and her labs showed a prepubertal estrogen level. Repeat bone age showed no further advancement. She continued to follow every 6 months for monitoring of her growth.

Clinical Pearls/Pitfalls

1. Estrogen-producing ovarian cyst should be considered in girls with isolated thelarche.
2. Simple ovarian cysts that autonomously produce estrogen tend to involute on their own without treatment; in most cases patients can be observed over time for resolution/regression of their GIPP.
3. Surgical referral is indicated for complex or large ovarian cysts.
4. GnRH agonists are not indicated in the treatment of GIPP.

Head Trauma

Case Presentation

A 5-year-old female is referred for breast development, pubic hair, and vaginal secretions. She was born full term to a healthy mother and had normal growth and development until age 4 years when the patient was a restrained passenger in a severe automobile accident. Sustaining multiple fractures and a closed head injury with depressed skull fractures, she was hospitalized for a prolonged period, including inpatient rehabilitation. She currently resides at home, though she has severe developmental delay and learning disabilities. Her home nurse noted breast and pubic hair development around 3–4 months ago and more recently saw whitish vaginal discharge in her diaper last month and once again last week. There is no pertinent family history and maternal menarche was at age 11 years.

On examination, her height is 109 cm (43 in.) at the 59th percentile and weight is 22 kg (48.5 lb) at the 89th percentile; BMI is 18.5 kg/m^2 at the 96th percentile. Her blood pressure is normal. She has no acne, hirsutism, or cutaneous findings. Pubertal status is Tanner stage 3 for breasts with estrogenization of aerolae. Pubic hair is Tanner 2. The vaginal mucosa appears slightly estrogenized. There is no clitoral enlargement.

Laboratory testing shows an FSH of 9.1 mIU/mL, LH of 4.5 mIU/mL, and estradiol of 25 pg/mL (range for prepubertal girls 5–20 pg/mL). Thyroid function is normal for age. Prolactin is 9 ng/mL (normal 3–24 ng/mL). Bone age X-ray is performed and read as consistent with the patient's chronologic age. Her most recent MRI, performed 1 month ago, shows generalized cortical atrophy, though a normal appearing pituitary.

Discussion

This patient has survived a traumatic brain injury (TBI) and now has signs of precocious puberty. Laboratory analysis shows a GDPP picture, similar to Case #1. GDPP resulting from TBI has been well described in the literature [38–42], though not completely well understood. The presumed mechanism of TBI-related PP is through the loss of hypothalamic inhibition of pituitary gonadotropins. Infundibular-hypophyseal structures are at particularly high risk of mechanical and vascular damage due to their anatomic placement and blood supply [28].

In a study of 31 children post-TBI, 29 % of patients had endocrine dysfunction at 12 months after injury, half of which showed precocious puberty [43]. In contrast, another study of 198 survivors of TBI, only 2 patients had precocious puberty, a rate consistent with the general population [44].

Beyond GDPP, patients with a history of TBI are at risk for other pituitary endocrine abnormalities, including growth hormone deficiency, central hypothyroidism, secondary adrenal insufficiency, and diabetes insipidus.

Management

The treatment of TBI-related GDPP is the same as idiopathic GDPP—with use of GnRH agonists to suppress the usual pulsatile action and subsequent gonadotropin release.

Outcome

This patient underwent placement of a histrelin implant. Repeat labs 3 months following the implantation showed improvement of gonadotropins and estradiol. Six months following the implantation, the breast development had completely regressed.

Clinical Pearls/Pitfalls

1. TBI brain injury may result in precocious puberty, as well as other endocrine abnormalities.
2. TBI-related precocious puberty is gonadotropin dependant.
3. The mechanism of this finding is not completely understood, but thought to be due to disinhibition of the pituitary gonadotropes at the level of the hypothalamus.
4. Treatment typically involves depot leuprolide acetate injections or long-acting yearly histrelin implantation.

Exogenous Hormones

Case Presentation

Two sisters, ages 4 and 7, are referred for breast development. Both girls are otherwise healthy, with the exception of eczema, treated with topical over-the-counter moisturizers. Their mother had noticed some breast development in her older daughter approximately 9 months ago and then in her younger daughter 4 months ago. She has not seen any axillary or pubic hair. There has been no vaginal bleeding, but mother is unsure about vaginal discharge. There is no family history of precocious puberty. Maternal menarche was at 14 years of age. The girls were both products of in vitro fertilization as the mother was 41 at the time of the first pregnancy and had difficulty conceiving; she is now menopausal.

On examination of the 7 year old, her height is 120 cm (47 in.) at the 37th percentile and weight is 31 kg (68 lb) at the 94th percentile; BMI is 21.5 kg/m^2 at the 98th percentile. Her blood pressure is normal. She has no acne, hirsutism, or cutaneous findings. Pubertal status is Tanner stage 3 for breasts with estrogenization of the aerolae. Pubic hair is Tanner 1. There is no axillary hair. The vaginal mucosa appears slightly pink. There is no clitoral enlargement.

On examination of the 4 year old, her height is 107 cm (42 in.) at the 91st percentile and weight is 17 kg (37 lb) at the 69th percentile; BMI is 14.8 kg/m^2 at the 35th percentile. Her blood pressure is normal. She has no acne, hirsutism, or cutaneous findings. Pubertal status is Tanner stage 2 for breasts with estrogenization of the aerolae. Pubic hair is Tanner 1. There is no axillary hair. The vaginal mucosa appears slightly pink. There is no clitoral enlargement.

Early morning laboratory testing on both girls shows low prepubertal gonadotropins and elevated estradiol (26 pg/mL for the 7 year old, 37 for the 4 year old). Adrenal androgens are prepubertal. 17-Hydroxyprogesterone is normal. Thyroid function was normal. Bone age X-rays are performed and read as slightly advanced for both girls. Pelvic ultrasound on both girls revealed normal ovaries without any masses or cysts.

Discussion

Examination and laboratory testing for these sisters shows a picture consistent with GIPP (low gonadotropins, elevated estradiol), though the ovaries appear normal on ultrasound. Prepubertal girls have an average ovarian size of 2.0 ± 1.5 cm^3 and by Tanner II, the average right ovarian size increases to 3.2 ± 3.0 cm^3 and 2.7 ± 1.8 cm^3 for the left ovary [45].

The fact that siblings developed the same condition at the same time should raise suspicions of an environmental factor. Exogenous estrogens can be found in multiple different places, from medications such as estrogen creams and oral contraceptive pills to contaminated foods, milk, from excessive drinking of soy formulas to many over the counter herbal remedies or multivitamins [46–49]. When taking a history with respect to precocious puberty, an astute clinician should inquire about exposures to other people's medications, herbal supplements or remedies, or other possible sources of exogenous estrogens.

Management

Upon removal or avoidance of the offending external source of estrogen, the symptoms should resolve and abate. Unfortunately, the source may not always be readily apparent and may require a detailed social, medical, and family history.

Outcome

Upon further questioning, it was discovered that the girls' mother has been using an estrogen cream, prescribed by her gynecologist. The girls, thinking that they were using a moisturizer for their eczema, were applying the estrogen cream to their skin when their parents were not watching them. Upon cessation of the cream, the girls' breast development regressed over the course of <6 months.

Clinical Pearls/Pitfalls

1. Exposure to exogenous estrogens can cause GIPP.
2. A careful history help along with traditional laboratory testing and imaging are useful tools to make this diagnosis.
3. Removal of the exposure will cause the signs and symptoms of precocious puberty to resolve.

Endocrine Disruptors

Case Presentation

A 6-year-old girl is referred for evaluation of pubic hair and breast development. She is recent immigrant to the United States, having moved here with her family from Colombia only 2 months prior. The family were farmers back in their home country, and the patient indicated that she misses being able to play in the fields all day with her father while he worked. She is otherwise healthy and has no other medical problems. She is developmentally appropriate and there is no significant family history.

On examination, her height is 125 cm (49 in.) at the 97th percentile and weight is 25 kg (55 lb) at the 89th percentile; BMI is 16 kg/m^2 at the 69th percentile. There are no prior growth records to review, but her midparental height is 64″. Her blood pressure is normal. She has no acne, hirsutism, or cutaneous findings. Breast development was Tanner stege 3 and pubic hair was Tanner stage 2. The vaginal mucosa was pink and physiologic discharge was present.

Early morning laboratory testing shows elevated gonadotropins (FSH 7 mIU/mL and LH 4.3 mIU/mL) and elevated estradiol of 40 pg/mL. Adrenal androgens are consistent with mid-puberty. 17-Hydroxyprogesterone is normal. Bone age X-ray is performed as read as advanced with a skeletal age of 10 years. MRI of the head/pituitary with and without contrast is performed and is normal. Further discussion reveals that the patient was likely chronically exposed to her father's pesticides while in the fields.

Discussion

Endocrine disruptors are environmental chemicals, either natural or manmade, that can interact with the normal hypothalamic–pituitary–gonadal axis [50–52]. In the case of female precocious puberty, this can be via directly binding to and activating estrogen receptors, by increasing aromatase activity, or through GnRH stimulation [53]. Therefore, PP due to endocrine disruptors may cause either GDPP or GIPP.

Phytoestrogens, such as daidzein, genistein, glycitein, and biochanin-A, are relatively weak estrogen mimetics and can be found naturally in certain foods. One would need to consume very large amounts of these foods—garlic, apple, legumes, and coffee—to see an observable estrogenic effect [54].

Synthetic endocrine disruptors are becoming increasingly cited as the cause for the ever-drifting lower age of the normal onset of puberty. These chemicals—diethylstilbestrol (DES), DDT, dioxin, and many other pesticides, industrial products, and compounds—have been implicated in affecting pubertal development in animal and human studies [35, 55]. DDT in particular, an organochlorine pesticide, can be biologically broken down into p,p′-DDE, a central disruptor of puberty. Though not commercially available in the United States and Europe since the 1970s, DDT is still used in developing countries worldwide [56]. Phthalates in plastics, including food containers, medical equipment, and children's toys, have been implicated in similar processes [57, 58].

Management

As with direct exogenous estrogen exposures, removal of the offending agent should improve the symptoms. Prior long-term chronic exposure to the agent, though, may result in the precocity taking a long time to resolve. Avoidance of PVC products and phthalate-containing plastics for play or food-storage should be maintained. If by removing the offending agent, the pubertal manifestations regress or stop progressing, no treatment is necessary. Although the mechanism underlying these cases of nonprogressive precocious puberty is unclear, it is known that the gonadotropic axis is not activated. In contrast, for cases in which precocious puberty progresses due to activation of the gonadotropic axis, removal of the offending agent does not result in regression of symptoms or arrest of progressive bone age advancement. In these cases, medical treatment with GnRH agonists may be indicated. In other cases, anti-estrogen or anti-androgen agents may be considered [50].

Outcome

After being exposure-free from DDT products, the patient's puberty did stop progressing, but due to such significant prior advancement in puberty, she was treated with histrelin (GnRH agonist) implant to prevent further progression of pubertal development.

Clinical Pearls/Pitfalls

1. Environmental compounds, either natural or manufactured, can cause disruption in the normal hypothalamic–pituitary–gonadal axis, resulting in precocious puberty.
2. A detailed history is necessary to decipher these difficult and varied disruptors.

References

1. Lee PA, Kulin HE, Guo SS. Age of puberty among girls and the diagnosis of precocious puberty. Pediatrics. 2001;107(6):1493.
2. Carel JC, Léger J. Clinical practice. Precocious puberty. N Engl J Med. 2008;358:2366.
3. Styne DM, Grumback MM. Puberty: ontogeny, neuroendocrinology, physiology, and disorders. In: Melmed S, Polonsky KS, Larsen PR, Kronenberg

HK, editors. Williams Textbook of Endocrinology. 12th ed. Philadelphia: Saunders Elsevier; 2011. p. 1054–201.

4. Kaplowitz PB, Oberfield SE. Reexamination of the age limit for defining when puberty is precocious in girls in the United States: implications for evaluation and treatment. Pediatrics. 1999;104:936–41.

5. Wu T, Mendola P, Buck GM. Ethnic differences in the presence of secondary sex characteristics and menarche among US girls: the Third National Health and Nutrition Examination Survey, 1988-1994. Pediatrics. 2002;110:752–7.

6. Kaplowitz PB, Slora EJ, Wasserman RC, Pedlow SE, Herman-Giddens ME. Earlier onset of puberty in girls: relation to increased body mass index and race. Pediatrics. 2011;108:347–53.

7. Rosenfeld RL, Cooke DW, Radovick S. Puberty and its disorders in the female. In: Sperling MA, editor. Pediatric Endocrinology. 3rd ed. Philadelphia: Saunders Elsevier; 2008. p. 530–609.

8. Banerjee S, Raghavan S, Wasserman EJ, Linder B, Saenger P, DiMartino-Nardi J. Hormonal findings in African-American and Caribbean Hispanic girls with premature adrenarche: implications for polycystic ovarian syndrome. Pediatrics. 1998;102:4.

9. DiMartino Nardi J. Premature adrenarche: findings in prepubertal African American and Caribbean Hispanic girls. Acta Paediatr Suppl. 1999;433:67–72.

10. Saenger P, Reiter EO. Premature adrenarche: a normal variant of puberty. (Editorial). J Clin Endocrinol Metab. 1992;74:236–8.

11. Ibáñez L, Potau N, Carrascosa A. Insulin resistance, premature adrenarche, and a risk of the polycystic ovary syndrome. Trends Endocrinol Metab. 1998;9(2):72–7.

12. Idkowiak J, Lavery GG, Dhir V, Barrett TG, Stewart PM, Krone N, Arlt W. Premature adrenarche: novel lessons from early onset androgen excess. Eur J Endocrinol. 2011;165(2):189–207.

13. Vuguin P, Saenger P, Dimartino-Nardi J. Fasting glucose insulin ratio: a useful measure of insulin resistance in girls with premature adrenarche. J Clin Endocrinol Metab. 2001;86(10):4618–21.

14. Vuguin P, Linder B, Rosenfeld RG, Saenger P, DiMartino-Nardi J. The roles of insulin sensitivity, insulin-like growth factor I (IGF-I), and IGF-binding protein-1 and -3 in the hyperandrogenism of African-American and Caribbean Hispanic girls with premature adrenarche. J Clin Endocrinol Metab. 1999;84(6):2037–42.

15. Kaplan SL, Grumbach MM. Pathogenesis of sexual precocity. In: Grumbach MM, Sizonenko PC, Aubert ML, editors. Control of the onset of puberty. Baltimore: Williams & Williams; 1990. p. 620–60.

16. Kotwal N, Yanamandra U, Menon AS, Nair V. Central precocious puberty due to hypothalamic hamartoma in a six-month-old infant girl. Ind J Endocrinol Metab. 2012;16(4):627–30.

17. Mittal S, Mittal M, Montes JL, Farmer JP, Andermann F. Hypothalamic hamartomas: part 1: clinical, neuroimaging, and neurophysiological characteristics. Neurosurg Focus. 2013;34(6), E6.

18. Mahachoklertwattana P, Kaplan S, Grumback M. The luteinizing hormone-releasing hormone-secreting hypothalamic hamartoma is a congenital malformation: natural history. J Clin Endocrinol Metab. 1993;77:118–24.

19. Jung H, Carmel P, Schwartz MS, Witkin JW, Bentele KH, Westphal M, Piatt JH, Costa ME, Cornea A, Ma YJ, Ojeda SR. Some hypothalamic hamartomas contain transforming growth factor alpha, a puberty-inducing growth factor, but not luteinizing hormone-releasing hormone neurons. J Clin Endocrinol Metab. 1999;84(12):4695–701.

20. Laue I, Comite F, Hench K, Loriaux D, Cutler CH, Pescovitz O. Precocious puberty associated with neurofibromatosis and optic gliomas. Am J Dis Child. 1985;139:1097.

21. Zacharin M. Precocious puberty in two children with neurofibromatosis type 1 in the absence of optic chiasmal glioma. J Pediatr. 1997;130:155–7.

22. Bridges NA, Cooke A, Healy MJ, et al. Ovaries in sexual precocity. Clin Endocrinol (Oxf). 1995;42:135–40.

23. Van Wyk JJ, Grumback MM. Syndrome of precocious menstruation and galactorrhea in juvenile hypothyroidism: an example of hormonal overlap in pituitary feedback. J Pediatr. 1960;57:416–35.

24. Buchanan CR, Stanhope R, Adlard P, et al. Gonadotropin, growth hormone and prolactin secretion in children with primary hypothyroidism. Clin Endocrinol (Oxf). 1988;29:427–36.

25. Hayward C, Killen JD, Wilson DM, Hammer LD, Litt IF, Kraemer HC, et al. Psychiatric risk associated with early puberty in adolescent girls. J Am Acad Child Adolesc Psychiatry. 1997;36:255–62.

26. Slap GB, Khalid N, Paikoff RL, Brooks-Gunn J, Warren MP. Evolving self-image, pubertal manifestations, and pubertal hormones: preliminary findings in young adolescent girls. J Adolesc Health. 1994;15:327–35.

27. Celio M, Karnik NS, Steiner H. Early maturation as a risk factor for aggression and delinquency in adolescent girls: a review. Int J Clin Pract. 2006;60:1254–62.

28. Sklar CA, Rothenberg S, Blumberg D, et al. Suppression of the pituitary-gonadal axis in children with central precocious puberty: effects on growth, growth hormone, insulin-like growth factor-1, and prolactin secretion. J Clin Endocrinol Metab. 1991;73:734–8.

29. Mittal S, Mittal M, Montes JL, Farmer JP, Andermann F. Hypothalamic hamartomas: surgical considerations and outcome. Neurosurg Focus. 2013;34(6):E7.

30. Chae HS, Rheu CH. Precocious pseudopuberty due to an autonomous ovarian follicular cyst: case report with a review of the literatures. BCM Res Notes. 2013;6:319.

31. Young RH, Dickerson GR, Scully RE. Juvenile granulose cell tumor of the ovary: a clinicopathologic analysis of 125 cases. Am J Surg Pathol. 1984;8:575–96.

32. Silverman LA, Gitelman SE. Immunoreactive inhibin, mullerian inhibitory substance, and activin as biochemical markers for juvenile granulosa cell tumors. J Pediatr. 1996;129:918–21.

33. Howell L, Bader A, Mullassery D, Losty P, Auth M, Kokai G. Sertoli Leydig cell ovarian tumour and gastric polyps as presenting features of Peutz-Jeghers syndrome. Pediatr Blood Cancer. 2010;55(1):206–7.

34. Millar DM, Blake JM, Stringer DA, Hara H, Babiak C. Prepubertal ovarian cyst formation:5 years' experience. Obstet Gynecol. 1993;81:434–8.

35. Tessiatore P, Guana R, Mussa A, Lonati L, Sberveglieri M, Ferrero L, Canavese F. When to operate on ovarian cysts in children? J Pediatr Endocrinol Metab. 2012;25(5-6):427–33.

36. Feuillan P, Calis K, Hill S, Shawker T, Robey PG, Collins MT. Letrozole treatment of precocious puberty in girls with the McCune-Albright syndrome: a pilot study. J Clin Endocrinol Metab. 2007;92:2100–6.

37. Eugster EA, Rubin SD, Reiter EO, Plourde P, Jou HC, Pescovitz OH. Tamoxifen treatment for precocious puberty in McCune-Albright syndrome: a multicenter trial. J Pediatr. 2003;143:60–6.

38. Sockalosky JJ, Kriel RL, Krach LE, Sheehan M. Precocious puberty after traumatic brain injury. J Pediatr. 1987;110(3):373–7.

39. Einaudi S, Matarazzo P, Peretta P, Grossetti R, et al. Hypothalamo-hypophysial dysfunction after traumatic brain injury in children and adolescents: a preliminary retrospective and prospective study. J Pediatr Endocrinol Metab. 2006;19(5):691–703.

40. Blendonohy PM, Philip PA. Precocious puberty in children after traumatic brain injury. Brain Inj. 1991;5(1):63–8.

41. Maxwell M, Karacostas D, Ellenbogen RG, Brzezinski A, et al. Precocious puberty following head injury: case report. J Neurosurg. 1990;73(1):123–9.

42. Shaul PW, Towbin RB, Chernausek SD. Precocious puberty following severe head trauma. Am J Dis Child. 1985;139(5):467–9.

43. Kaulfers AM, Backeljauw PF, Reifschneider K, Blum S, Michaud L, Weiss M, Rose SR. Endocrine dysfunction following traumatic brain injury in children. J Pediatr. 2010;157(6):894–9.

44. Heather NL, Jefferies C, Hofman PL, Derraik JG, et al. Permanent hypopituitarism is rare after structural traumatic brain injury in early childhood. J Clin Endocrinol Metab. 2012;97(2):599–604.

45. Razzaghy-Azar M, Ghasemi F, Hallaji F, Ghasemi A, Ghasemi M. Sonographic measurement of uterus and ovaries in premenarcheal healthy girls between 6 and 13 years old: correlation with age and pubertal status. J Clin Ultrasound. 2011;39(2):64–73.

46. Partsch CJ, Sippell WG. Pathogenesis and epidemiology of precocious puberty. Effects of exogenous oestrogens. Hum Reprod Update. 2001;7(3):292–302.

47. Aksglaede L, Juul A, Leffers H, Skakkebaek NE, Andersson AM. The sensitivity of the child to sex steroids: possible impact of exogenous estrogens. Hum Reprod Update. 2006;12(4):341–9.

48. Maruyama K, Oshima T, Ohyama K. Exposure to exogenous estrogen through intake of commercial milk produced from pregnant cows. Pediatr Int. 2010;52:33–8.

49. Andersson AM, Skakkebæk NE. Exposure to exogenous estrogens in food: possible impact on human development and health. Eur J Endocrinol. 1999;140:477–85.

50. Buck Louis GM, Gray LE, Marcus M, Ojeda SR, Pescovitz OH, et al. Environmental factors and puberty timing: expert panel research needs. Pediatrics. 2008;121:192–207.

51. Cesario SK, Hughes LA. Precocious puberty: a comprehensive review of literature. J Obstet Gynecol Neonatal Nurs. 2007;36(3):263–74.

52. Özen S, Goksen D, Darcan Ş. Agricultural pesticides and precocious puberty. Vitam Horm. 2014;94:27–40.

53. Özen S, Darcan Ş. Effects of environmental endocrine disruptors on pubertal development. J Clin Res Pediatr Endocrinol. 2011;3(1):1–6.

54. Roy JR, Chakraborty S, Chakraborty TR. Estrogen-like endocrine disrupting chemicals affecting puberty in humans—a review. Med Sci Monit. 2009;15:137–45.

55. Abaci A, Demir K, Bober E, Buyukgebiz A. Endocrine disruptors with special emphasis on sexual development. Pediatr Endocrinol Rev. 2009;6: 464–75.

56. Krstevska-Konstantinova M, Charlier C, Craen M, DuCaju M, Heinrichs C, de Beaufort C. Sexual precocity after immigration from developing countries to Belgium: evidence of previous exposure to organochlorine pesticides. Hum Reprod. 2001;16:1020–6.

57. Jobling S, Reynolds T, White R, Parker M, Sumpter J. A variety of environmentally persistent chemicals, including some phthalate plasticizers, are weakly estrogenic. Environ Health Persp. 1995;103:582–7.

58. Blount B, Silva M, Caudill S, Needham L, Pirkle J, Sampson E, et al. Levels of seven urinary phthalate metabolites in a human reference population. Environ Health Perspect. 2000;108:979–82.

Chapter 3
Constitutional Delay of Growth and Puberty

M. Tracy Bekx and Ellen Lancon Connor

Abbreviations

ALS	Acid labile subunit
CDGP	Constitutional delay of growth and puberty
FSH	Follicle-stimulating hormone
GnRH	Gonadotropin-releasing hormone
HH	Hypogonadotropic hypogonadism
IGF1	Insulin-like growth factor
IGFBP3IGF	Binding protein 3
LH	Luteinizing hormone
MPH	Mid-parental prediction of height
PAH	Predicted adult height

M.T. Bekx, M.D. (✉) • E.L. Connor, M.D.
Division of Pediatric Endocrinology, University of Wisconsin,
600 Highland Avenue, H4/4, Madison, WI 53792, USA
e-mail: mtbekx@pediatrics.wisc.edu; elconnor@pediatrics.wisc.edu

© Springer International Publishing Switzerland 2016
H.L. Appelbaum (ed.), *Abnormal Female Puberty*,
DOI 10.1007/978-3-319-27225-2_3

Introduction

The girl with constitutional delay of puberty and growth (CDGP) represents one end of the spectrum of the normal pubertal timing and linear growth of childhood. Genetically programmed to have a slowdown of linear growth as a toddler, with subsequent bone age delay but normal childhood growth velocity, the girl with constitutional delay will by definition eventually have a normal pubertal growth spurt, normal pubertal development, and a final adult height appropriate for her family's genetic potential, albeit at an age significantly older than her female peers. The practitioner is obligated to distinguish girls with CDGP from hypothalamic and pituitary disorders preventing puberty, as well as from gonadal failure.

To be defined as having constitutional delay of growth and puberty, a girl should have

1. A history of growth velocity slowing between 18 and 36 months of age
2. Normal growth velocity after 3 years of age
3. A delayed bone age for chronological age and sex
4. Pubertal delay more than 2–2.5 standard deviations from the mean

Pubertal delay has traditionally been defined as the lack of thelarche by the age of 13 years or the lack of menarche by the age of 15 years. Most girls with CDGP will also have a first degree relative with a history consistent with CDGP. However, autosomal recessive, X-linked, and sporadic forms have also been described [1]. Therefore, a girl could have CDGP without having a parent with a history of CDGP. Furthermore, if a girl is adopted, family history may not be available.

Case Presentation

A 13 and 8/12 years old girl was seen in clinic complaining of lack of breast budding and lack of menarche. She is a healthy girl who has been growing at third percentile for height and weight since age

3 years. She had a birth weight at 50th percentile and birth length at 40th percentile. Mid-parental height is 29th percentile. Review of systems is negative for all findings except lack of pubertal development. Family history is positive for a father who grew 4 in. in college and began shaving at age 21 years, and an older sister who had a similar growth pattern and is now at the 22nd percentile for height after menarche at age 16.5 years. Physical examination reveals a girl who appears younger than stated age and is not dysmorphic. Breasts are Tanner 1. No pubic hair is present. Bone age radiograph is 10 years.

Discussion

Genetics

Family pedigree analysis has suggested that constitutional delay is inherited in an autosomal dominant fashion most commonly but may also exist in X-linked and autosomal recessive forms. Monozygotic twin studies point to considerable homogeneity in pubertal timing as well. CDGP heritability accounts for 50–80 % of pubertal onset variability (Banerjee 2007). A number of candidate genes have been suggested. Genetic analysis of affected individuals identified leptin gene mutations in one pedigree, and GH secretagogue receptor GHSR mutations in another. A region of Chromosome 2 has been suggested for other gene mutation analysis [2]. Gene mutations in the ALS gene have been postulated but not yet identified [3]. Gonadotropin-releasing hormone (GnRH) defects were suspected, but at least one analysis found these defects in patients with idiopathic hypogonadotropic hypogonadism but not CDGP [4].

A heterozygous novel missense variant in the leptin gene, which occurs at chromosome 7pq13, was identified in a boy with delayed puberty due to CDGP, a slim body habitus (commonly seen in CDGP), and reduced appetite and also in his mother who had the identical phenotype with a history of menarche at age 15 years [5]. Thirty one patients with CDGP were studied for growth hormone secretagogue receptor (GHSR) mutations, as well as 65 patients with idiopathic short stature, and in 150 adults and 197 children with normal stature. GHSR binds ghrelin and two females with CDGP were found to have a unique mutation that resulted in ghrelin secretion; they both had delayed puberty and ultimately, normal adult heights [2].

Fifty-two families affected by CDGP were studied via linkage analysis in Finland. This method detected a pericentromeric region of Chromosome 2 that predisposed to pubertal delay. The region involved was chromosome 2p13–2q13. Authors postulated a gene affecting the timing of pubertal onset [2].

A British study examined a possible link of the acid labile subunit (ALS) to CDGP. ALS binds insulin-like growth factor (IGF1) and IGF binding protein 3 (IGFBP3) in circulation to stabilize the complex. The IGFALS gene is found on Chromosome 16. Individual case reports had described ALS mutations in single patients who had short stature and mildly delayed puberty, but not family history of CDGP. Ninety children with CDGP were studied; none were found to have mutations of IGFALS [3].

Thus, the current state of knowledge is that CDGP is frequently heritable, but the genetic factor responsible is usually unknown. Therefore, genetic analysis for a CDGP gene in most families as a diagnostic confirmation is not standard of practice. However, knowledge of a positive family history of CDGP can be helpful in identifying a young girl who will also have CDGP.

Distinguishing CDGP from Other Forms of Short Stature

The practitioner seeing a young girl with possible CDGP must identify whether another cause could explain delayed puberty and short stature. Possible causes of the pubertal delay can be separated into those having ovarian origin (hypergonadotropic hypogonadism) versus those having central nervous system origin (hypogonadotropic hypogonadism). A short statured girl with ovarian failure would most likely be manifesting signs of Turner syndrome or gonadal dysgenesis, two of the more common causes of hypergonadotropic hypogonadism. Other causes include more rare genetic syndromes, galactosemia, radiation and chemotherapy, infection, and pelvic trauma. By contrast, the differential diagnosis of causes for poor growth and hypogonadotrophic hypogonadism is lengthy and includes (1) many types of chronic disease involving various organ systems, (2) hypothalamic or pituitary disease, tumor, or malformation, (3) genetic variations of gonadotropin function, and (4) malnutrition, including eating disorders. The normal variant of CDGP is sometimes considered a mild familial variant of temporary hypogonadotropic hypogonadism that will resolve without intervention.

Judicious use of history, review of systems, reconstructed growth chart, physical examination, and bone age radiograph will allow the practitioner to begin to discriminate among the many causes of delayed puberty and to assess which girls need laboratory evaluations. In those girls needing further study, the history, ROS, and exam will usually provide clues as to which laboratory evaluations should be sought. Given the large role of heritability in CDGP, family history can be particularly helpful. However, for those girls with sporadic or recessive forms of CDGP, history may not be conclusive.

Evaluation

The complete physical exam is important, with focus on features suggestive of an underlying syndrome or disease, as well as puberty staging. For example, findings suspicious for Turner syndrome include downslanting palpebral fissures, posteriorly rotated ears, webbed neck, broad chest, wide carrying angle of arms, pitted nails, and shortened limbs with increased upper to lower body segment proportions. Assessment of the ovarian contribution to puberty includes breast development by Tanner staging. Clinical findings suggestive of androgen production (body odor, axillary hair, and pubic hair production) may occur independent of ovarian contribution, reflecting adrenal activation. Adrenarche may occur without thelarche in Turner syndrome and thelarche may occur without adrenarche in androgen insensitivity syndrome. By contrast, a girl with CDGP will have either no pubertal changes, or pubertal changes consistent with an age much younger than her chronological age (consistent with her bone age).

Constitutional delay of growth and puberty (CDGP) is a normal and commonly encountered variant of growth. For girls brought to medical attention, the chief concern is the absence of thelarche by age 13 years, as well as short stature and/or attenuation of growth. The clinician's job is to determine if the girl has a normal variant of growth (CDGP), or underlying pathology contributing to growth attenuation and delayed puberty. CDGP, hypogonadotropic hypogonadism (functional or permanent), or hypergonadotropic hypogonadism may present with short stature and lack of pubertal findings. An initial step in assessment is a reconstruction of the girl's growth story, from infancy, when nutrition is a key player in linear growth, through childhood, when growth hormone and genetics play the larger role. In CDGP, a pattern of significant growth attenuation occurs in the transition between infancy and childhood, followed by return to normal growth velocity, albeit at a lower height percentile (Fig. 3.1).

Birth history should include birth weight and length, and inquiry regarding maternal complications during the pregnancy, such as diabetes, smoking, hypertension, or poor growth in utero. The majority of infants born small for gestational age (SGA), birth weight, and/or length less than 2 SDS below the mean for their gestational age and sex, demonstrate catch up growth, however, some do not [6]. Those with in utero growth retardation (IUGR) may have an underlying genetic syndrome that can impact both growth and pubertal onset, for example, Turner syndrome or Russell Silver syndrome. Turner syndrome, due to the absence of part or all of one X chromosome, may present with left-sided congenital heart defects, carpal and pedal edema, small stature, webbing of the neck, low posterior hairline, frequent otitis media, and primary ovarian failure. Russell Silver syndrome may present with lack of appetite, failure to thrive, triangular facies, limb hemihypertrophy, clinodactyly, and precocious puberty.

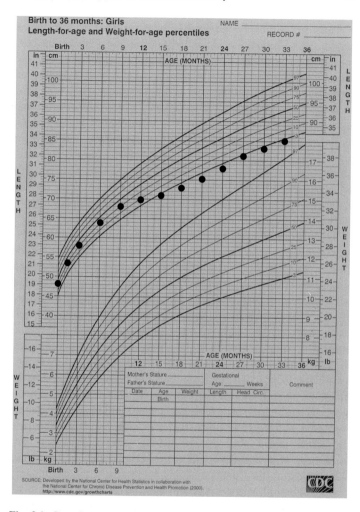

Fig. 3.1 Growth curve of birth to 36 months of age in toddler with CDGP demonstrating slowing of growth by age 18 months, followed by eventual normal growth velocity, but at a lower length percentile

Past medical history can identify factors that impact growth and stature. These factors include underlying chronic illnesses, medication use, and screening for evolving health concerns. Some examples are cystic fibrosis, chronic renal disease, poorly controlled diabetes, and use of medications such as steroids (that can suppress growth) or stimulants for ADHD (which can suppress appetite and temporarily inhibit linear growth) [7]. History of poor weight gain or failure to thrive can strongly influence growth and onset of puberty. Examples include undiagnosed celiac disease or anorexia nervosa, or even an unstable home environment, leading to psychosocial failure to thrive. Finally, concerns of anosmia may suggest Kallmann syndrome, with permanent hypogonadotropic hypogonadism (Fig. 3.2).

The history of extended family members' final adult heights, growth patterns, and pubertal onset is important to determine if growth is normal for the family pattern and plays a key role in supporting the diagnosis of CDGP. A strong tendency of delayed puberty (onset of menarche after age 14 years in females, or history of a pubertal growth spurt after age 16 years of age males) is consistent with CDGP. Likewise, the mid-parental height (MPH), an estimate of a child's genetic height potential using parents' heights, should be calculated to determine if current growth pattern is reasonably anticipated given family genetics (Table 3.1). The MPH should be plotted, and the percentile at which it rests at adulthood noted. This should be used to determine the child's corrected height percentile using current height and the bone age rather than the chronologic age.

If there is a significant disparity between the mother's and father's heights, the calculated target height may not be reliable.

Calculating growth velocity and plotting on the available CDC growth velocity curves for gender is an important element in assessing normal growth. Growth velocity reaches its nadir prior to onset of puberty, reflecting the transition to sex steroid-driven growth. This period of slow growth is followed by a rise and peak in growth velocity during puberty, on average for girls at an age of 11.5 years (8.3 cm/year) in North America [8]. Those with CDGP often show declining height percentiles on the growth curve at these chronologic ages, as peers are experiencing acceleration in growth velocity (Fig. 3.3).

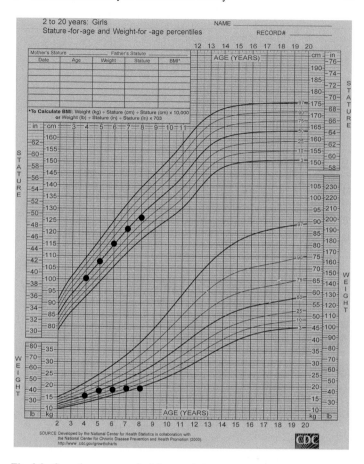

Fig. 3.2 Growth curve seen in failure to thrive

Table 3.1 Calculating mid-parental height (MPH) in centimeters

Girls	(Mom's height + (Dad's height−13 cm))/2
Boys	(Dad's height + (Mom's height + 13 cm))/2

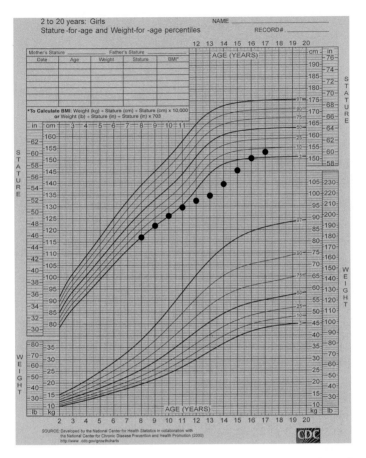

Fig. 3.3 Growth curve in child with CDGP, demonstrating slowing of growth near average timing of puberty, followed by growth acceleration later, mirroring the later onset of puberty

Management

Diagnosis

Initial laboratory evaluation should be based upon findings from the history and physical examination, as well as growth curves. Evaluation may include chronic disease screening for anemia, underlying renal or hepatic disease, celiac disease, inflammatory bowel disease, and thyroid dysfunction. Screening luteinizing hormone (LH), follicle-stimulating hormone (FSH), and estradiol should be obtained in all girls with delayed puberty to evaluate for evidence of ovarian failure or lack of CNS stimulation of the ovaries. Baseline growth hormone markers, including IGF-1 and IGFBP-3, should be obtained in short statured girls with delayed puberty if growth velocity is abnormal. Elevated FSH and LH levels, consistent with hypergonadotropic hypogonadism, should be further evaluated with karyotype and further investigation for causes of primary gonadal failure.

A bone age radiograph, to assess the skeletal maturation, by sequence of and distinct changes in ossification centers, and ultimate closure of epiphyses, is central to diagnosis of CDGP. The Greulich–Pyle Atlas or Tanner–Whitehouse method is used commonly in determining bone age, matching and scoring similar appearing bones to a "standard" [9] In CDGP, this reading is delayed (usually up to 2–3 years), which is congruent with delayed onset of puberty. The bone age is also an important tool in assessing the predicted adult height (PAH), comparing the delay in bone age relative to chronologic age as a marker of growth potential. The most common method applied is the Bayley–Pinneau method, which utilizes tables for predicting adult height from skeletal age, based on the Greulich–Pyle hand standards [10]. This is most reliable in children with normal growth and may be less reliable in other situations.

A challenge in girls with possible CDGP, who are otherwise appear healthy, is distinguishing CDGP from permanent hypogonadotropic hypogonadism (HH). Features suggestive of CDGP include a strong family history of delayed puberty with eventual normal final height and spontaneous puberty, whereas evidence of anosmia or hyposmia, familial pubertal delay requiring medical intervention, or a history of CNS lesions or injury supports the diagnosis of HH. Baseline gonadotropins are low in both and GnRH stimulation testing results can be overlapping, with a positive pubertal response defined as a predominant LH response over FSH following GnRH stimulation testing, or an LH > 5–8 IU/L, depending on the assay used [11, 12]. The majority of studies investigating this conundrum focus on males with no significant published data in girls, and none have demonstrated a test with 100 % sensitivity or specificity. The gold standard is time and observation, with eventual progression into puberty for those with CDGP no later than age 18 years.

Girls with a delayed bone age and low IGF-1 levels, who continue to demonstrate a decline in growth velocity, should be tested for growth hormone deficiency by a growth hormone stimulation test. Levels greater than 10 ng/mL indicate adequate growth hormone secretion [13]. In girls with low stimulated growth hormone levels, pituitary magnetic resonance imaging is important to assess for anatomic abnormalities, such as tumors, or an ectopic/hypoplastic gland.

In summary, the diagnostic evaluation of the girl presenting with delayed puberty and growth attenuation involves a thorough review of her growth history, past medical history, family history, and assessment for underlying causes. Often in CDGP the girl's evaluation will reveal normal growth velocity after the age of 3 years, delayed bone age and positive family history for delayed puberty (Table 3.2).

Therapeutic Options

When CDGP is diagnosed in a girl, the ensuing question is how to proceed and whether any intervention is warranted. Many factors affect this decision, including her current age, anticipated timing of puberty based on family history, and psychosocial concerns. For those that are at greater extremes (significant short stature or delayed puberty), a greater impetus to intervene may exist.

Oxandrolone in Girls with CDGD

One of the medical options of treatment for CDGP is oxandrolone. This oral medication is a weak nonaromatizable androgen that stimulates growth and has minimal impact on growth plate

Table 3.2 Assessment of delayed puberty and growth attenuation

Growth history	Birth length and weight
	Maternal complications during pregnancy
	Review of growth charts, including weight
	Assessment of growth velocity
Family history	Parents' heights
	Parents' timing of puberty
	Extended family members' heights and timing of puberty
Medical history	Underlying chronic disease medications
Physical exam	Syndromic features
	Evidence of estrogenization (thelarche)
	Assess sense of smell
Laboratory considerations	CBC with differential
	ESR
	Basic Metabolic Panel
	Liver function tests
	Celiac screen
	Thyroid studies
	IGF-1 and IGFBP-3
	LH, FSH, and estradiol
	Karyotype—if concerns of hypergonadotropic hypogonadism
Radiology	Bone age
	MRI of pituitary if evidence of growth hormone deficiency

maturation in children with bone ages >8 years. Oxandrolone's effects on growth, although not completely understood, are felt to be independent of growth hormone, as IGF-1 levels remain unchanged when measured during therapy [14, 15].

For young girls, the majority of studies examining effects of oxandrolone therapy on growth have been in Turner syndrome, and very few have been in girls with CDGP. The use of oxandrolone in Turner syndrome has been studied for many years for optimizing stature [16]. Results are consistently positive in demonstrating increases in growth velocity and final height [16, 17]. Major side effects are uncommon but generally dose related/androgen related and include increased acne, deepening of voice, and clitoromegaly, all disconcerting when present in a young adolescent girl. A summary of recent publications assessed efficacy and safety of oxandrolone in Turner syndrome, specifically addressing the effects of medication dosing on gains in growth velocity versus side effects. In this review, all three main studies demonstrated an increase in growth velocity and gain in final adult height with the addition of oxandrolone to growth hormone treatment (2.3–4.6 cm gain). The major concerns of dose-related side effects included voice deepening, hirsutism, and clitoromegaly. In addition, there were concerns of delayed breast development despite the addition of supplemental estrogen and a decrease in HDL. Whether the effects on breast are due to underlying factors in Turner syndrome were not explored. The authors' recommendations for oxandrolone therapy in the Turner syndrome population include: initiating therapy after age 8 years of age, using an optimal dose of 0.03–0.05 mg/kg/day with a maximum dose of 2.5 mg a day, along with proper counseling and reduction of dosing if side effects present [18].

Studies looking specifically at the use of oxandrolone in girls with CDGP are few, and thus much of the clinical decision to prescribe is based on experience in boys with CDGP and the use of oxandrolone in select female populations. If oxandrolone is prescribed for girls with confirmed CDGP, it should be at a low dose, and patients and families need to be counseled on the risks of androgen effects.

Estrogen and Girls with CDGP

One of the defining features of CDGP is the later pubertal onset. For some girls, this delay in development can be emotionally and socially difficult.

Sex hormone therapy may be prescribed at low doses for girls with CDGP to address the absence of pubertal signs, although published studies are scarce. Wehkalampi et al. looked at the use of low-dose estrogen to promote final height in girls with CDGP. In this cohort, 7 of 39 girls received low-dose estrogen using an estradiol gel (17B-estradiol 0.1–0.6 mg per day) or weekly patch (12.5–50 µg per week, which corresponds to 0.1–0.4 mg of 17B-estradiol per day). Therapy started at a mean age of 13.5 years for a mean duration of 2.5 years. No differences in age at acceleration, age of peak height velocity, age of menarche, pubertal height gain, or adult height were noted. The addition of low-dose estrogen did not reduce or increase final adult height. How the addition of estrogen impacted quality of life and self-esteem was not explored [19].

For estrogen replacement in adolescent girls, the recommendation is the use of the transdermal route to promote the greatest benefit on growth and puberty with the least risk of side effects [20]. Studies of the effects of oral versus transdermal estrogen therapy in those with hypopituitarism and on growth hormone therapy showed a greater decline in insulin-like growth factor 1 levels (IGF-1) with oral versus transdermal estrogen replacement [21, 22]. Similarly, studies of estrogen replacement in Turner syndrome demonstrated that transdermal and intramuscular estrogen replacement therapy had a better outcome on final adult height than oral replacement [23]. Transdermal estrogen avoids hepatic first pass effect, thus potentially lowering the risk of thrombogenicity or adverse effect on lipids.

In summary, low-dose transdermal estrogen may be used in the treatment of girls with CDGP to stimulate onset of puberty and growth acceleration. Care should be taken to avoid accelerating bone age advancement. The decision to treat should include a discussion with the patient and family of goals of therapy and expectations of final adult height. Bone age must be followed closely to prevent undue loss of height potential.

Prognosis of Girls with CDGP

As CDGP is a normal variant of growth, the long-term prognosis is generally good for overall health and fertility. For final adult height in girls with CDGP, published data is minimal. Studies in boys show that mean final height is often lower than both mid-parental height and predicted adult height, and is influenced by factors including height deficit prior to onset of puberty, earlier timing of significant growth attenuation, and shorter growth spurt [24]. Predicting those girls, who will be most severely affected, remains difficult.

Wekhalampi et al. examined the growth patterns and final adult heights in 39 girls with a history of CDGP and compared it to their genetic target height. The data revealed a mean final height within the population mean and near the mean target height, although nearly half of the girls had final adult heights more than 0.5 SDS below their target height and 15 % had an adult height great than 1 SDS below the target height. As seen with boys, the height deficit was greatest in those that demonstrated a decreased in height SDS in earlier childhood between ages of 3 and 8 years, as opposed to those whose growth was more affected later in childhood [19].

Similar findings were described in a cohort of girls with CDGP defined as no thelarche by age 13 years, bone age delayed by more than 1.5 years, no clinical evidence of chronic disease, and normal karyotype [25]. Height SDS score improved from a mean height SDS score of −3.4 to a final height SDS of −1.5. The final height was closer to the predicted adult height based on bone age assessment, but this calculation varied, consistent with the observation that accurate height predictions are difficult in the individual patient. This study also failed to demonstrate differences in self-esteem (versus "normal" height), marital status or stable relationships, or employment [25].

For young girls with CDGP, there may be acute psychosocial concerns of delayed puberty, being incongruent from peers in terms of sexual development. Interestingly, there is no evidence of increased depression in girls with delayed puberty. A systematic review with a meta-analysis of four cohort studies evaluated the effects of pubertal timing in girls and incidence of depression and found no increased risk of depression in those with delayed puberty [26].

Outcome in Case Report

The patient was counseled regarding the likely diagnosis of CDGP given her family history, growth curves, physical findings, and bone age radiograph. She was also counseled regarding the likelihood that thelarche would ensue soon, given her current bone age. She and her parents elected not to seek pharmaceutical intervention but to "wait and watch." At a 6 months follow-up visit, thelarche was noted with breasts bilaterally Tanner 2. A second follow-up visit 9 months from the initial consultation documented linear growth acceleration and the appearance of a few terminal pubic hairs along the center of the labia majora, with continued progression of breast development. Menarche occurred at age 16 years 6 months. At age 17 years, a repeat bone age was 15 years, and she was estimated to be near final height. Her final height was at the 20th percentile, and menses were occurring at intervals of 32 days.

In summary, most girls with CDGP eventually reach an expected reasonable height based on family patterns and proceed through puberty, with no long-term consequences in health, fertility, or quality of life. Appropriate counseling of girls with CDGP and parents may alleviate fears and acute concerns.

Clinical Pearls and Pitfalls

1. Family history should be elicited in evaluating girls with apparent delayed puberty.
2. Girls with CDGP will have a delayed bone age and a prepubertal normal growth velocity. Most girls with CDGP will also have a family history of CDGP.
3. CDGP does not require intervention for a height outcome that is congruent with family history.
4. CDGP will result in normal puberty occurring at a later age than typical for girls and at a height that is generally consistent with the height percentile of the mid-parental height.

References

1. Banerjee I, Clayton P. The genetic basis for the timing of human puberty. J Neuroendocrinol. 2007;19:831–8.
2. Pugliese-Pires PN, Fortin JP, Arthur T, Latronico AC, et al. Novel inactivating mutations in the GH secretagogue receptor gene in patients with

constitutional delay of growth and puberty. Eur J Endocrinol. 2011;165: 233–41.

 3. Banerjee I, Hanson D, Perveen R, Whatmore A, Black GC, Clayton PE. Constitutional delay of growth and puberty is not commonly associated with mutations in the acid labile subunit gene. Eur J Endocrinol. 2008;158:473–7.

 4. Beneduzzi D, Trarbach EB, Min L, Jorge AAL, et al. Role of gonadotro-pin-releasing hormone receptor mutations in patients with a wide spectrum of pubertal delay. Endocr Dev. 2014;102(3):838–46.

 5. Murray PG, Read A, Banerjee I, Whatmore A, et al. Reduced appetite and body mass index with delayed puberty in a mother and son: association with a rare novel sequence variant in the leptin gene. Eur J Endocrinol. 2011;164:521–7.

 6. Clayton PE, Cianfarani S, Czernichow P, Johannsson G, Rapaport R, Rogal A. Management of the child born small for gestational age through to adulthood: a consensus statement of the International Societies of Pediatric Endocrinology and the Growth Hormone Research Society. J Clin Endocrinol Metab. 2007;92:804–10.

 7. Harstad EB, Weaver AL, Katusic SK, Colligan RC, Kumar S, Chan E, Voigt RG, Barbaresi WJ. ADHD, stimulant treatment, and growth: a longi-tudinal study. Pediatrics. 2014;134(6):e935–44.

 8. Abassi V. Growth and normal puberty. Pediatrics. 1998;102(2 Pt3): 507–11.

 9. Gilli G. The assessment of skeletal maturation. Horm Res. 1996;45 Suppl 2:49–52.

10. Bramswig JH, Fasse M, Holthoff ML, et al. Adult height in boys and girls with untreated constitutional delay of growth and puberty, accuracy of five different methods of height prediction. J Pediatr. 1990;117(6):886–91.

11. Harrington J, Palmert MR. Distinguishing constitutional delay of growth and puberty from isolated hypogonadotropic hypogonadism: critical appraisal of available diagnostic tests. J Clin Endocrinol Metab. 2012;97:3056–67.

12. Palmert MR, Dunkel L. Delayed puberty. N Engl J Med. 2012;366: 443–53.

13. Allen DB, Cuttler LC. Short stature in childhood-challenges and choices. N Engl J Med. 2013;368:1220–8.

14. Kaplowitz P. Delayed puberty. Pediatr Rev. 2010;31(5):189–95.

15. Vottero A, Pedori S, Verna M, Pagaono B, Cappa M, Loche S, Bernasconi S, Ghizzoni L. Final height in girls with central idiopathic precocious puberty treated with gonadotropin-releasing hormone analog and oxandro-lone. J Clin Endocrinol Metab. 2006;91:1284–7.

16. Nilsson KO, Albertsson-Wikland K, Alm J, Aronson S, Gustafsson J, Hagenas L, Hager A, Ivarsson SA, Karlberg J, Kristrom B, Marcus C, Moell C, Ritzen M, Tuvemo T, Wattsgard D, Westgren U, Westphal O, Aman J. Improved final height in girls with Turner's Syndrome treated with growth hormone and oxandrolone. J Clin Endocrinol Metab. 1996;81:635–40.

17. Stahnke N, Keller E, Landy H, Serona Study Group. Favorable final height outcome in girls with Ullrich-Turner syndrome treated with low-dose growth hormone together with oxandrolone despite starting treatment after 10 years of age. J Pediatr Endocrinol Metab. 2002;15:129–38.
18. Sas TC, Gault EJ, Bardsley MZ, Menke LA, Freriks K, Perry RJ, Otten BJ, de Muinck Keizer-Schrama SM, Timmers H, Wit JM, Ross JL, Donaldson MD. Safety and efficacy of oxandrolone in growth hormone-treated girls with turner syndrome: evidence from recent studies and recommendations for use. Horm Res Paediatr. 2014;81:289–97.
19. Wehkalampi K, Päkklia K, Laine T, Dunkel L. Adult height in girls with delayed pubertal growth. Horm Res Paediatr. 2011;76:130–5.
20. Dunkel L, Quinton R. Transition in endocrinology: induction of puberty. Eur J Endocrinol. 2014;170:R229–39.
21. Phelan N, Conway SH, Llahana S, Conway GS. Quantification of the adverse effect of ethinylestradiol containing oral contraceptive pills when used in conjunction with growth hormone replacement in routine practice. Clin Endocrinol (Oxf). 2012;76:729–33.
22. van der Klaauw AA, Biermasz NR, Zelissen PM, Pereira AM, Lentjes EG, Smit JW, van Thiel SW, Romijn JA, Roelfsema F. Administration route-dependent effects of estrogens on IGF-1 levels during fixed GH replacement in women with hypopituitarism. Eur J Endocrinol. 2007;157:709–16.
23. Davenport ML. Evidence of early initiation of growth hormone and trans-dermal estradiol therapies in girls with Turner syndrome. Growth Horm IGF Res. 2006;16(Suppl A):S91–7.
24. Poyrazuglu S, Günöz H, Darendeliler F, Saka N, Bundak R, Bas F. Constitutional delay of growth and puberty: from presentation to final height. J Pediatr Endocrinol Metab. 2005;18:171–9.
25. Crowne EC, Shalet SM, Wallace WH, Eminson DM, Price DA. Final height in girls with untreated constitutional delay in growth and puberty. Eur J Pediatr. 1991;150(10):712.
26. Galvao TF, Silva MR, Zimmermann IR, Souza KM, Martins SS, Pereira MG. Pubertal timing in girls and depression: a systematic review. J Affect Disord. 2014;155:13–9.

Chapter 4
Premature Ovarian Failure

Amit Lahoti, Lakha Prasannan, and Phyllis W. Speiser

Abbreviations

AMH	Anti-mullerian hormone
DHEAS	Dehydroepiandrosterone sulfate
DSD	Disorders of sex development
DXA	Dual energy X-ray absorptiometry

A. Lahoti, M.D.
Division of Pediatric Endocrinology, Le Bonheur Children's Hospital,
University of Tennessee Health Science Center,
Memphis, TN, USA

Department of Obstetrics and Gynecology, Northwell Health System,
Hofstra Northwell School of Medicine, Hempstead, NY, USA

L. Prasannan, M.D.
Department of Obstetrics and Gynecology, Northwell Health System,
Hofstra Northwell School of Medicine, Hempstead, NY, USA

P.W. Speiser, M.D. (✉)
Division of Pediatric Endocrinology, Cohen Children's
Medical Center of NY, 1991 Marcus Avenue, Ste M100,
Lake Success, NY 11042, USA

Hofstra Northwell School of Medicine,
Hempstead, NY, USA
e-mail: pspeiser@nshs.edu

© Springer International Publishing Switzerland 2016
H.L. Appelbaum (ed.), *Abnormal Female Puberty*,
DOI 10.1007/978-3-319-27225-2_4

FSH   Follicular stimulating hormone
LH   Luteinizing hormone
OMIM   Online Mendelian Inheritance in Man
POF   Premature ovarian failure
rhGH   Recombinant hormone growth hormone
TS   Turner syndrome
TSH   Thyroid stimulating hormone

Introduction

Premature ovarian failure (POF) is a heterogeneous disorder
defined as amenorrhea and hypergonadotropic hypogonadism
before age 40 years. Onset at an earlier age can present with
delayed puberty or interruption of pubertal progression. Lack of
breast development by the age of 13 or failure of menarche to
occur by age 15 may be indications of POF. This condition must be
differentiated from several other causes of delayed or interrupted
puberty or amenorrhea. The diagnosis of POF is often associated
with physiological and psychological consequences. A detailed
history including birth history, prior medical history, and family
history can provide valuable information. Physical examination
focusing on pubertal staging and identification of associated dysmorphic features or genital ambiguity should guide further laboratory and/or radiological investigations. Timely diagnosis and
management of ovarian failure is essential to prevent additional
physiological and psychological sequelae. In addition, anticipatory
counseling, screening for, and management of, comorbidities will
likely improve overall quality of life of these patients.

Case Presentation #1

A 8.8-year-old girl was referred for evaluation for short stature in
the setting of Turner syndrome (TS; karyotype: 45,X) diagnosed
by amniocentesis performed for advanced maternal age. Aside
from a slight hearing deficit treated with speech therapy, she was

in good health. Her growth plotted on a standard CDC growth chart (see Fig. 4.1) showed that height had been at the 10–25 % up to the age of 5.5 years, but subsequently decreased gradually to the 3 % by the time she was referred at age 8 years. Birth weight was 2.8 kg. Mid-parent height was 63 inches (corresponding to ~25 %

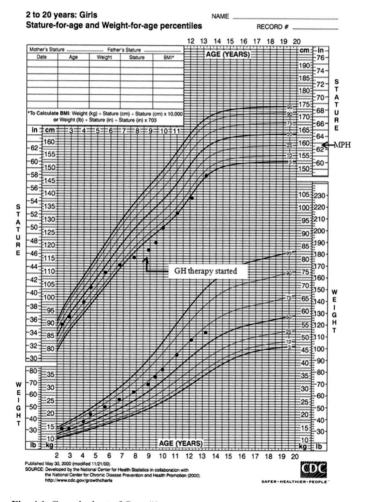

Fig. 4.1 Growth chart of Case #1

on a standard CDC growth chart). Weight was steady at 50–75 %. Review of systems, family and social histories were unremarkable. She was described as a gifted student.

Physical examination at her initial visit showed height at 3 %, weight at 74 %, and BMI at 95 %. Vital signs were notable for normal blood pressure and heart rate. She appeared husky, proportional, and had subtle but recognizable dysmorphic features, including low set ears and short left 5th metacarpal. Examination of various organ systems including head, eyes, ears, nose and throat, cardiovascular, respiratory, abdominal, extremities, and neurological system was normal. She had no thyroid enlargement. She had a hypopigmented macule on the back, which was diagnosed as vitiligo. Breast and pubic hair distribution was consistent with Tanner stage 1.

Initial evaluation for organic causes of growth failure showed normal thyroid function, insulin-like growth factor-1 (IGF-1) and insulin-like growth factor binding protein-3 (IGFBP-3) levels; and negative serologic screening tests for celiac disease, inflammatory bowel disease, or any other chronic systemic diseases.

She did not start puberty spontaneously, and laboratory evaluation at 11 years age showed LH and FSH >50 mIU/mL, estradiol at 10 ng/dL indicating ovarian failure.

Case Presentation #2

A 15-year-old girl with a history of ataxia telangiectasia and cerebral palsy presented with amenorrhea. She began to have breast development at 9 years and occasional vaginal spotting for 1½ years. She was not sexually active, and there was no history of caloric restriction or excessive exercise. There was no nipple discharge, psychotropic drug use, or other related symptoms.

On examination, her breasts and pubic hair were Tanner stage 4. The abdominal examination was benign with no masses and no tenderness. The external genitalia were normal and the lower one-third of the vagina was visualized in the frog-legged position with gentle traction of the labia and noted to be normal. There was no vaginal bleeding.

Laboratory evaluation included serum testosterone, dehydroepiandrosterone sulfate (DHEAS), prolactin, thyroid-stimulating hormone (TSH) and tissue transglutaminase IgA and IgG, which were all normal. Serum estradiol: 14 ng/dL (low), FSH: 55.7 IU/L, and LH: 51.5 IU/L (both markedly elevated). PCR for fragile X was negative. Karyotype showed 46, XX, inv [14] (q13q24) (paracentric inversion of chromosome 14 with breakpoints at bands 14q13 and 14q24). Pelvic ultrasound identified a 5.2 cm uterus. The right ovary measured 2.3 × 2.0 × 1.5 cm and the left ovary measured 3.1 × 2.7 × 3.4 cm. Patient was diagnosed with arrest of pubertal development secondary to early ovarian failure.

Discussion

Interruption or lack of pubertal development along with laboratory findings of hypergonadotropic hypogonadism (elevated gonadotropins and low estradiol level) represents the most severe presentation of POF. Similarly, POF can present with delayed or prolonged puberty, but more commonly, POF is associated with secondary amenorrhea. POF affects 1/10,000 women by age 20, 1/1000 women by age 30 years and 1/100 women by age 40 years (prevalence of 1 %) [2]. While the underlying cause of POF remains unknown in up to 90 % of cases, the identified causes of POF are extremely heterogeneous and include both genetic and acquired causes [3, 4] (see Table 4.1).

In at least 10–15 % of patients with premature ovarian failure, a genetic cause has been determined [4]. Genetic causes related to defects in sex chromosomes include X-chromosome aneuploidy-like monosomy, trisomy X, and X-chromosome rearrangements. Both the short and long arms of X-chromosome appear to contain important genes for ovarian function. Specific X-chromosome gene defects that have been associated with POF or gonadal dysgenesis include *BMP15, FMR1, and FMR2.* Fragile X carrier screening is recommended for women of all ages with POF. Premutations of the FMR1 gene are the most common genetic cause of POF [5]. The degree of ovarian dysfunction depends on CGG repeat length (CGG repeats between 55 and 200 in the FMR1 gene increases risk of POF), although the relationship is not linear [6]. FMR1-related POF occurs in approximately 21 % of females who have an FMR1 premutation, and these women may experience earlier menopause by approximately 5 years. Due to potential repeat instability upon transmission of premutation alleles, women with alleles in this range are considered to be at risk of having children affected with fragile X syndrome [7].

Several autosomal genes have also been associated with POF. While these include some syndromic causes as listed in Table 4.1; other identified causes include polymorphisms and mutations involving isolated genes including *INHA, FOXL2, FOXO3,* and those for LH, FSH, and estrogen receptors *(LHR, FSHR, and ER alpha)* [2]. Recently, a homozygous deletion in the gene-encoding stromal antigen 3 (*STAG3*) on chromosome 7 has been identified as a cause for POF. *STAG3* encodes a subunit of *cohesin,* a large protein complex that is essential for proper pairing and segregation of chromosomes during meiosis. The deletion results in a severely truncated protein and early meiotic arrest. Human *STAG3* expression is found to be restricted to early meiosis in fetal ovaries in females, with those affected noting to be sterile, and their fetal oocytes arrested at early prophase I, leading to oocyte depletion at 1 week of age [8]. Patients with disorders of sexual differentiation (DSD) where the genotype and phenotype are discordant may have female or ambiguous appearing external genitalia and a 46,XY karyotype. In conditions with complete or partial gonadal dysgenesis due to gene mutations like *MAP3K1 or SF1 (latter also associated with sex reversal),* the dysgenetic gonads fail to function resulting in subsequent absence of spontaneous pubertal development [9].

Ataxia telangiectasia (AT) is an autosomal recessive disorder caused by homozygous or compound heterozygous mutation in ATM gene on chromosome 11q22 which predisposes patients to chromosomal breakage. Typical clinical features include cerebellar ataxia, telangiectasias, immune defects, and a predisposition to malignancies. Ovarian dysfunction and POF is one of the

Table 4.1 Known causes of premature ovarian failure (POF)

Genetic causes	Acquired causes
Sex chromosome abnormalities	**Iatrogenic**
• Turner syndrome (TS)	• Surgery, exposure to chemotherapeutic agents (e.g., alkylating agents), radiation therapy
• Fragile X pre-mutation carriers (*FMR1* gene), OMIM entry #309550	**Autoimmune**
• X chromosome deletions, inversions, duplications and translocations	• Autoimmune polyglandular syndrome type I and II
Autosomal gene abnormalities	• Autoimmune lymphocytic opphoritis
• Galactosemia, OMIM entry #230400	**Infections**
• Blepharophimosis-ptosis-epicanthus inversus syndrome (BPES), OMIM entry #110100	• Herpes zoster, cytomegalovirus, Mumps, etc.
• Perrault syndrome, OMIM entry #233400	**Toxins**
• Ataxia telangiectasia, OMIM entry #208900	• Candidate environmental ovotoxicants include: polycyclic aromatic hydrocarbons (PAHs), carbamates, etc. [39]
• Bloom syndrome (BLM), OMIM entry #210900	• Iron overload
• Pseudohypoparathyroidism (PHP) type Ia, OMIM entry #103580	
• Isolated gene defects like: follicle stimulating hormone (FSH) receptor (FSHR) mutations, luteinizing hormone (LH) receptor (LHR) mutations, mutation in the eukaryotic translation initiation factor 4E nuclear import factor 1, *STAG3, FIGL4, NOBOX*	
• Steroidogenic enzyme defects: CYP17 deficiency, StAR mutation, Aromatase gene mutations	
• Intraovarian modulators: BMP15, polymorphisms of inhibin alpha subunit	
• Disorders of sexual differentiation (DSD)	

OMIM Online Mendelian Inheritance in Man

Source: Hamosh A, Scott AF, Amberger JS. Online Mendelian Inheritance in Man (OMIM), a knowledgebase of human genes and genetic disorders. Nucleic Acids Res. 2005: D514–7

comorbidities that have been described in these patients [4, 10]. However, due to the rarity of this condition, the etio-pathogenesis is not completely clear. The patient in Case #2 also had a paracentric inversion of chromosome 14, a finding not unusual in ataxia telangiectasia [11], although its role in causing POF is not known. In the future, microarray or whole exome sequencing may help further define the genetic cause of POF in AT.

Turner syndrome (TS) accounts for 50–60 % of patients with gonadal dysgenesis, and hence is an important cause of POF. This disorder is characterized by the absence of all or part of the X-chromosome and occurs in 1 in 2500 to 1 in 3000 live-born girls [12, 13]. The karyotype in approximately half of patients is monosomy X (45,X). Molecular studies have shown that the maternal X is retained in two-thirds of patients with TS and the paternal X in the remaining one-third [14]. The remainder may have mosaicism for 45,X, with 1 or more additional cell lineages (including those with Y chromosome), or have an isochromosome X with duplication of long arm of X chromosome i(Xq) [13]. In patients who have a demonstrable chromosome aberration, the karyotype–phenotype correlations show that the aberration common to all those with the complete TS is monosomy of loci on short arm of the X-chromosome [15].

Cardinal features seen in TS include short stature, webbed neck, widely spaced nipples, streak gonads, and associated congenital auditory and/or cardiovascular malformations. Cardiovascular anomalies including coarctation of the aorta, renal anomalies, hearing impairment, otitis media and mastoiditis, congenital lymphedema and an increased incidence of hypertension, achlorhydria, diabetes mellitus, and Hashimoto thyroiditis have all been identified in this patient population [12, 15, 16]. Some patients are diagnosed as newborns due to congenital lymphedema of the hands and feet or redundant nuchal skin. However, most are diagnosed in adolescence years as they fail to enter puberty or fail to develop secondary sexual characteristics. Many TS patients lack specific dysmorphic features described above. These patients present with short stature, poor breast development, and primary amenorrhea [12].

Short stature may be the only apparent clinical finding initially, and it is the only phenotypic abnormality present in virtually 100 %

of patients with a 45,X karyotype. Monosomy of the short arm of the X-chromosome with deletion or mutation of SHOX is the decisive factor in the causation of short stature and congenital malformations in TS. Therefore, karyotype testing should be considered in children and adolescents with height below the third percentile [17].

In most girls with TS, ovaries contain normal numbers of primordial germ cells for up to at least 6 weeks of gestation, but at later gestational ages, the numbers of germ cells are decreased and replaced by a white fibrous streak, which will not secrete appropriate sex steroid hormones. Studies indicate that gonadal dysgenesis may be caused by accelerated apoptosis, rather than abnormal germ cell formation [17]. Histologically, the streak gonad is characterized by interlacing waves of dense fibrous stroma, indistinguishable from normal ovarian stroma. Of note, the uterus and vagina are normal and capable of responding to exogenous hormones. Therefore, when ovarian atresia is incomplete, pubertal changes, spontaneous menstruation, and even pregnancies have been reported. The incidence of spontaneous puberty in TS is reported to be between 5 and 10 % and, more recently in some series, as high as 20 % among mosaic TS patients [18].

Autoimmune lymphocytic oophoritis, a known specific cause of premature ovarian failure, was first described in association with Addison disease and adrenal autoimmunity [19]. There is also a strong association between POF and autoimmune polyendocrine syndromes (both type I and type II). This condition may include hypothyroidism, adrenal insufficiency, hypoparathyroidism, and type 1 diabetes mellitus [6]. However, POF has also been described in women with non-endocrine autoimmune disorders such as myasthenia gravis, rheumatoid arthritis, or systemic lupus erythematosus [5]. The exact mechanism that causes the initiation of ovarian autoimmunity is essentially unknown. It may be triggered by various agents: viruses, bacteria, or ovarian self-antigens [20].

There are several clinical features that are unique to autoimmune oophoritis. A striking characteristic of autoimmune oophoritis is sparing of primordial follicles and cortex of the ovary. Theca cells of the developing follicles are predominantly infiltrated by mononuclear inflammatory cells [19, 21]. These women are also noted to have significantly larger ovarian volumes with a polycystic appearance as determined by sonographic examination. The cystic formation is hypothesized to be due to the elevated levels of gonadotropins [19, 21, 22]. There is also a presence of antiadrenal antibodies (and often primary adrenal insufficiency), though the signs and symptoms of POF typically precede the development of adrenal insufficiency in women with autoimmune oophoritis by several years [19].

Anti-adrenal antibody titers represent a more sensitive test for ovarian autoimmunity compared with anti-ovarian antibodies [6]. This is done by the measurement of steroidogenic cell autoantibodies, especially anti-21-hydroxylase antibodies, by immunoprecipitation assay. It is considered essentially equivalent to measurement of adrenal cortex autoantibodies by immunofluorescence. There is no known immunosuppressive therapy for autoimmune oophoritis that has been proven safe and effective by a prospective randomized placebo-controlled study [19].

A number of inherited enzymatic pathway disorders have been associated with ovarian follicular dysfunction leading to POF. Classic galactosemia, an inherited disorder caused by Galactose 1-phosphate uridyl transferase (GALT) deficiency was one of the first to be characterized [6]. POF occurs in almost all women homozygous for mutations in the GALT gene that nearly or completely abolish GALT activity and are associated with a severe phenotype. Overall 17–67 % galactosemic women are reported to have POF. Histologically, ovaries in affected young women revealed severely decreased number of primordial follicles with normal morphology, without intermediate or mature follicles. In their teens and twenties, ovaries have been found to be hypoplastic and streak-like, suggesting developmental arrest [5, 23].

Etiology and timing of this disturbance in follicle development: whether prenatal, chronic postnatal, or a combination of both is not yet clear [5, 23]. It is theorized that ovarian damage develops due to the accumulation of galactose and its toxic metabolites (galactose-I-phosphate and galactitol) after birth. Apart from this, aberrant glycosylation of glycoproteins or glycolipids, UDP-galactose deficiency causing apoptosis of oocytes and ovarian stromal cells may also result in follicular dysfunction [5, 23].

Because galactosemia requires treatment in childhood to prevent mental retardation, it is unlikely to be diagnosed in an otherwise healthy adult presenting only with POF [5]. Treatment with a galactose-restricted diet is paramount to prevent mental retardation but despite early diagnosis and dietary intervention, independent complications such as ovarian dysfunction with subsequent infertility can occur [23]. There is currently no treatment for prevention of ovarian dysfunction in these patients; however, once diagnosed management is similar to POF from other causes.

Exposure to excess iron (iron overload) either due to hereditary causes (hereditary hemochromatosis) or due to chronic transfusions (as in beta-thalassemia, aplastic anemia) is known to cause hypogonadism due to pituitary iron deposition. There may also be a component of direct effects of iron and oxidative stress on the ovaries [24].

Management

Diagnostic evaluation is dictated by the clinical presentation. However, the most commonly performed initial tests include measurement of serum LH, FSH, and estradiol. FSH level is usually greater than 30 mIU/mL and suggests ovarian failure. A pelvic ultrasound to evaluate internal reproductive organs should also be performed. Pelvic ultrasound in patients with Turner syndrome and other causes of gonadal dysgenesis may be unable to detect ovaries or may demonstrates dysgenetic or streak ovaries. In some cases, the ovaries may appear structurally normal on ultrasound. Ultrasound will also be useful in evaluating abnormalities of uterus and cervix as well as to evaluate the thickness of the endometrial stripe. A karyotype to evaluate for sex chromosome aneuploidy or structural abnormalities of chromosomes is recommended. Karyotyping during evaluation of POF may also identify a previously undiagnosed DSD. Fragile X carrier screening is recommended for all girls with POF.

Antibodies to steroid 21 hydroxylase should be measured to exclude autoimmune oophoritis. Measurement of urine/serum

HCG and serum TSH, T4, and prolactin may be measured to exclude pregnancy, hypothyroidism, and hyperprolactinemia, respectively. Anti-mullerian hormone (AMH) in peripheral circulation is primarily derived from antral follicles (which reflect the primordial follicle pool). Hence, AMH may be an indirect measure of the ovarian reserve [25]. AMH level less than 1.0 ng/mL reflects diminished ovarian reserve. However, while very low AMH levels may be an early sign of impending POF or ovarian insufficiency, further research is needed to evaluate the predictive value of very low AMH levels [4]. AMH levels are also increasingly studied as markers of fertility and success of advanced reproductive techniques (ART). The results of a recent meta-analysis showed that in women undergoing ART, AMH has some association with implantation and clinical pregnancy but its predictive ability is weak. The predictive accuracy for clinical pregnancy was somewhat better for women with diminished ovarian reserve although this subgroup included older women and did not specifically study women with premature ovarian failure [26]. TS patients who do achieve spontaneous puberty and those with a fair probability of fertility (based on karyotype, e.g., mosaic TS 45,X/46,XX) appear to have higher AMH levels than other TS patients. Furthermore, in TS patients, AMH levels have been correlated with the number of follicles in biopsied ovarian tissue [25]. AMH continues to be a promising marker for clinical evaluation of future fertility; however, more studies are needed before AMH can be used to make clinical decisions in patients with POF.

Adolescents with POF will require hormone replacement therapy to induce and maintain secondary sexual characteristics. In prepubertal patients, the goal of estrogen replacement is to induce timely pubertal increases in the size of breasts and uterus and replicate a tempo of puberty, growth, and timing of menarche comparable to peers. However, as in patients with TS, some-times, in order to strike a balance between growth and puberty, hormone replacement and menarche may have to be delayed while the young girl is first treated with growth hormone to enhance height. Estrogen replacement is preferentially provided by micronized 17-beta estradiol (E_2) via oral or transdermal routes. Estradiol is identical to the ovarian product and the most physiological form of estrogen currently available. Oral estrogen undergoes first pass metabolism in liver leading to a higher serum estrone concentration, while transdermal preparations do not have this effect [27, 28]. Transdermal preparations can provide smaller estrogen doses. Several regimens of transdermal estradiol are clinically used and no single regimen has been shown to be better than others due to the absence of randomized-controlled trials in this field. However, most experts recommend individualizing the regimen beginning at age 11–12 years and progressing gradually. The dot matrix type of estradiol patch can also be cut in halves and quarters allowing for beginning estradiol concentrations as low as 6–7 µg with an increase in dose every several months based on clinical response and a goal to achieve adult replacement doses over 2–3 years of therapy [29]. Once full estrogen replacement doses are reached, cyclical progesterone as medroxyprogesterone acetate (5–10 mg) or micronized progesterone (200–400 mg) daily can be added for 10–12 days per month to induce menstrual bleeding. Cyclic therapy with estrogen-progesterone may be given with combined oral contraceptives, although even the low-dose estrogen–progesterone combination pills supply much larger amounts of estrogen than are delivered by transdermal estrogen therapy. When full replacement doses have been reached, the oral preparations may offer advantages in the form of simplicity of regimen.

Though the optimal age for initiation of rhGH in patients with TS has not been established, treatment should typically be considered when the height falls below the fifth percentile for age [12]. Non-aromatizable anabolic steroid, such as oxandrolone (dose of 0.05 mg/kg per day or less) has been tried as an adjunct therapeutic agent in those TS patients with extreme short stature with some promising results, though this use is not a standard practice as yet [30, 31].

If an underlying secondary cause is identified for POF, treatment for the specific diagnosis may require additional treatment and/or subspecialist referral. For example, patients with autoimmune oophoritis need to be screened for other autoimmune diseases especially autoimmune adrenal insufficiency and thyroid disease, which if present, need to be appropriately treated by an endocrinologist. If a patient is found to have hemochromatosis as the cause for ovarian insufficiency, she should be referred to a hematologist for consideration of iron chelation and screening for other effects of iron overload.

Since peak bone density is reached in mid-20s, osteoporosis is a serious concern for patients with POF especially those affected at an early age. Estrogen and progesterone replacement begun at puberty and continued until the expected age of menopause assists in completing adolescent bone maturation and optimizing peak bone mass. In addition, patients should be screened for vitamin D deficiency by measuring 25-OH vitamin D [25(OH)D] levels. While data on optimum 25(OH)D levels required to maintain normal bone density is somewhat lacking, many experts recommend dietary or supplemental vitamin D intake to keep levels >30 ng/mL [32]. Adequate dietary or supplemental calcium intake (about 1000 mg of elemental calcium daily in the preteen years and 1200–1500 mg daily after 11 years of age), as well as weight-bearing exercise should also be encouraged [12]. If patients develop osteoporosis, other specific treatments may be required.

After a diagnosis of POF is made, in addition to the hormone replacement treatment, patients also require long-term surveillance, management, and counseling for other sequelae including infertility and negative effects on neurological, psychological, cardiovascular, and skeletal health. Baseline dual energy X-ray absorptiometry (DXA) scan should be obtained to evaluate bone mineral density. As per current standards, DXA results for children are reported as areal bone mineral density (aBMD) Z-score. These scores are SD(s) based on the mean aBMD for the patient's chronological age and sex. Although T-scores are often automatically generated in DXA report, they should not be used for individuals who have not attained peak bone mass (usually by age 20 years, but may be even later in some patients with POF). Significant short stature, growth delay, and delay in puberty are factors that impact interpretation of aBMD. While mathematical corrections are not available for all of these variables, it is important to take these factors into consideration when interpreting aBMD *Z*-score measurements that are based on comparison to controls with average timing of growth and puberty [33]. Evidence-based guidelines for how often should DXA be monitored are lacking and there is a need for prospective studies; however, monitoring bone density every 2 years may be reasonable [29].

Transdermal estrogen replacement therapy was begun at age 12 years, and our patients were treated with gradually increasing doses, starting with a fractional 25 μg transdermal estrogen patch, until the full adult dose of 100 μg transdermal patch was attained. Breast enlargement occurred over time. Two years after initiation of estrogen, oral progesterone was added to for 10 days of each month to protect the endometrium from the hyperplastic effects of unopposed estrogen and to induce menses.

Outcomes

For the patient with TS (Case #1), rhGH therapy was discontinued at 14 years age when she reached adult height of 60 in. Both patients were also advised to take supplemental vitamin D and calcium at the diagnosis of POF. The DXA scan done at 13 years age showed low normal bone density in hip and spine (age-matched *Z*-score: spine −0.4, hip: −1.4). DXA scan results were not available for Case #2 as she was lost to follow-up. The TS patient will continue to be followed in concert with a cardiologist and nephrologist and undergo hearing tests as per clinical guidelines [12].

Fertility counseling will be addressed at future visits. Approximately 5–10 % of patients diagnosed with POF may conceive spontaneously and unexpectedly after their diagnosis [34]. The appropriate age for employing ART for this population of patients is not standardized and may be complicated by the psychological impact of the procedures and consent issues. Furthermore, when evaluating fertility options, the underlying etiology for POF should be taken into consideration and comorbidities must be addressed. For example, patients with TS may have cardiovascular and/or renal disease that can complicate a pregnancy. A cardiovascular evaluation is extremely important prior to considering ART because the risk of aortic dissection or rupture during pregnancy in a TS patient may be 2 % or higher than the general population which can increase the mortality for these patients by as much as 100-fold. Additionally, women with TS can have aortic dissection during pregnancy even without aortic root dilation [5].

In prepubertal girls who do not have mature eggs, ovarian tissue cryopreservation (OTC) technologies may be possible, though this technique for preservation of fertility is still experimental. The challenge in OTC lies in developing methods to support the maturation of the primordial follicles in order that they will produce mature, fertilizable oocytes. Several approaches have been investigated, including autotransplantation and in vitro maturation (IVM). Of these, only autotransplantation of cryopreserved tissue has been shown to result in live human births to date [35, 36]. Alternative methods of assisted reproduction include utilizing donor eggs. The cumulative chance of pregnancy after four IVF cycles using donor oocytes is close to 90 % [37]. In cases where ovarian preservation or ovum donation is not possible, adoption may be a reasonable option [38].

Clinical Pearls/Pitfalls

1. POF should be suspected in adolescents with abnormal pubertal progression and elevated gonadotropins.
2. Patients with Turner syndrome, disorders of sexual differentiation (DSD), and other syndromes associated with POF should have periodic screening for gonadal failure.
3. Screening for Fragile X premutation and karyotyping should be considered in all patients with premature ovarian failure.
4. Prompt diagnosis and institution of hormone replacement therapy will help initiate or restore physical development.
5. Fertility options should be discussed with a reproductive specialist at the time of diagnosis.
6. Patients with POF due to autoimmunity should undergo periodic screening for other autoimmune disorders.

References

1. Neely EKF, Fechner PY, Rosenfeld RG. Turner syndrome. In: Lifshitz F, editor. Pediatric endocrinology, Volume 2. 5th ed. New York: Informa Healthcare; 2009: p. 305–24.
2. Cordts EB, Christofolini DM, Dos Santos AA, Bianco B, Barbosa CP. Genetic aspects of premature ovarian failure: a literature review. Arch Gynecol Obstet. 2011;283(3):635–43.
3. Beck-Peccoz P, Persani L. Premature ovarian failure. Orphanet J Rare Dis. 2006;1:9.
4. Kovanci E, Schutt AK. Premature ovarian failure: clinical presentation and treatment. Obstet Gynecol Clin North Am. 2015;42(1):153–61.
5. Jin M, Yu Y, Huang H. An update on primary ovarian insufficiency. Sci China Life Sci. 2012;55(8):677–86.
6. Cox L, Liu JH. Primary ovarian insufficiency: an update. Int J Women's Health. 2014;6:235–43.
7. Saul RA, Tarleton JC. FMR1-Related Disorders. In: Pagon RA, Adam MP, Ardinger HH, Wallace SE, Amemiya A, Bean LJH, et al., editors. GeneReviews(R). Seattle, WA; 2012; accessed online 12/24/15.
8. Caburet S, Arboleda VA, Llano E, Overbeek PA, Barbero JL, Oka K, et al. Mutant cohesin in premature ovarian failure. N Engl J Med. 2014;370(10):943–9.
9. Baxter RM, Arboleda VA, Lee H, Barseghyan H, Adam MP, Fechner PY, et al. Exome sequencing for the diagnosis of 46, XY disorders of sex development. J Clin Endocrinol Metab. 2015;100(2):E333–44.
10. Miller ME, Chatten J. Ovarian changes in ataxia telangiectasia. Acta Paediatr Scand. 1967;56(5):559–61.
11. Aurias A, Dutrillaux B, Buriot D, Lejeune J. High frequencies of inversions and translocations of chromosomes 7 and 14 in ataxia telangiectasia. Mutat Res. 1980;69(2):369–74.
12. Bondy CA. Turner syndrome study G. Care of girls and women with Turner syndrome: a guideline of the Turner Syndrome Study Group. J Clin Endocrinol Metab. 2007;92(1):10–25.
13. Gravholt CH. Epidemiological, endocrine and metabolic features in Turner syndrome. Eur J Endocrinol. 2004;151(6):657–87.
14. Mathur A, Stekol L, Schatz D, MacLaren NK, Scott ML, Lippe B. The parental origin of the single X chromosome in Turner syndrome: lack of correlation with parental age or clinical phenotype. Am J Hum Genet. 1991;48(4):682–6.
15. Ferguson-Smith MA. Karyotype-phenotype correlations in gonadal dysgenesis and their bearing on the pathogenesis of malformations. J Med Genet. 1965;2(2):142–55.
16. Carr DH. Chromosome studies in spontaneous abortions. Obstet Gynecol. 1965;26:308–26.

17. Singh RP, Carr DH. The anatomy and histology of XO human embryos and fetuses. Anat Rec. 1966;155(3):369–83.

18. Pasquino AM, Passeri F, Pucarelli I, Segni M, Municchi G. Spontaneous pubertal development in Turner's syndrome. Italian Study Group for Turner's syndrome. J Clin Endocrinol Metab. 1997;82(6):1810–3.

19. Bakalov VK, Anasti JN, Calis KA, Vanderhoof VH, Premkumar A, Chen S, et al. Autoimmune oophoritis as a mechanism of follicular dysfunction in women with 46, XX spontaneous premature ovarian failure. Fertil Steril. 2005;84(4):958–65.

20. Shamilova NN, Marchenko LA, Dolgushina NV, Zaletaev DV, Sukhikh GT. The role of genetic and autoimmune factors in premature ovarian failure. J Assist Reprod Genet. 2013;30(5):617–22.

21. Hoek A, Schoemaker J, Drexhage HA. Premature ovarian failure and ovarian autoimmunity. Endocr Rev. 1997;18(1):107–34.

22. Lonsdale RN, Roberts PF, Trowell JE. Autoimmune oophoritis associated with polycystic ovaries. Histopathology. 1991;19(1):77–81.

23. Rubio-Gozalbo ME, Gubbels CS, Bakker JA, Menheere PP, Wodzig WK, Land JA. Gonadal function in male and female patients with classic galactosemia. Hum Reprod Update. 2010;16(2):177–88.

24. Roussou P, Tsagarakis NJ, Kountouras D, Livadas S, Diamanti-Kandarakis E. Beta-thalassemia major and female fertility: the role of iron and iron-induced oxidative stress. Anemia. 2013;2013:617204.

25. Broer SL, Broekmans FJ, Laven JS, Fauser BC. Anti-Mullerian hormone: ovarian reserve testing and its potential clinical implications. Hum Reprod Update. 2014;20(5):688–701.

26. Tal R, Tal O, Seifer BJ, Seifer DB. Antimullerian hormone as predictor of implantation and clinical pregnancy after assisted conception: a systematic review and meta-analysis. Fertil Steril. 2015;103(1):119–30. e3.

27. Gonzalez L, Witchel SF. The patient with Turner syndrome: puberty and medical management concerns. Fertil Steril. 2012;98(4):780–6.

28. Torres-Santiago L, Mericq V, Taboada M, Unanue N, Klein KO, Singh R, et al. Metabolic effects of oral versus transdermal 17beta-estradiol (E(2)): a randomized clinical trial in girls with Turner syndrome. J Clin Endocrinol Metab. 2013;98(7):2716–24.

29. Committee opinion no. 605: primary ovarian insufficiency in adolescents and young women. Obstet Gynecol. 2014;124(1):193–7.

30. Rosenfeld RG, Attie KM, Frane J, Brasel JA, Burstein S, Cara JF, et al. Growth hormone therapy of Turner's syndrome: beneficial effect on adult height. J Pediatr. 1998;132(2):319–24.

31. Gault EJ, Perry RJ, Cole TJ, Casey S, Paterson WF, Hindmarsh PC, et al. Effect of oxandrolone and timing of pubertal induction on final height in Turner's syndrome: randomised, double blind, placebo controlled trial. BMJ. 2011;342:d1980.

32. Holick MF, Binkley NC, Bischoff-Ferrari HA, Gordon CM, Hanley DA, Heaney RP, et al. Evaluation, treatment, and prevention of vitamin D

deficiency: an Endocrine Society clinical practice guideline. J Clin Endocrinol Metab. 2011;96(7):1911–30.

33. Crabtree NJ, Arabi A, Bachrach LK, Fewtrell M, El-Hajj Fuleihan G, Kecskemethy HH, et al. Dual-energy X-ray absorptiometry interpretation and reporting in children and adolescents: the revised 2013 ISCD Pediatric Official positions. J Clin Densitom. 2014;17(2):225–42.

34. Nelson LM, Covington SN, Rebar RW. An update: spontaneous premature ovarian failure is not an early menopause. Fertil Steril. 2005;83(5):1327–32.

35. Gracia CR, Chang J, Kondapalli L, Prewitt M, Carlson CA, Mattei P, et al. Ovarian tissue cryopreservation for fertility preservation in cancer patients: successful establishment and feasibility of a multidisciplinary collaboration. J Assist Reprod Genet. 2012;29(6):495–502.

36. West ER, Zelinski MB, Kondapalli LA, Gracia C, Chang J, Coutifaris C, et al. Preserving female fertility following cancer treatment: current options and future possibilities. Pediatr Blood Cancer. 2009;53(2):289–95.

37. Paulson RJ, Hatch IE, Lobo RA, Sauer MV. Cumulative conception and live birth rates after oocyte donation: implications regarding endometrial receptivity. Hum Reprod. 1997;12(4):835–9.

38. Hirshfeld-Cytron J, Gracia C, Woodruff TK. Nonmalignant diseases and treatments associated with primary ovarian failure: an expanded role for fertility preservation. J Women's Health. 2011;20(10):1467–77.

39. Iorio R, Castellucci A, Ventriglia G, Teoli F, Cellini V, Macchiarelli G, et al. Ovarian toxicity: from environmental exposure to chemotherapy. Curr Pharm Des. 2014;20(34):5388–97.

Chapter 5
Endocrine Disorders and Delayed Puberty

Allison Bauman, Laura Novello, and Paula Kreitzer

Abbreviations

ACTH	Adrenocorticotropic hormone
ART	Assisted reproductive technology
BMI	Body mass index
CBC	Complete blood count
CMP	Comprehensive Metabolic Panel
DHEAS	Dehydroepiandrosterone sulfate
FSH	Follicle stimulating hormone
GnRH	Gonadotropin-releasing hormone

A. Bauman, D.O. • L. Novello, M.D.
Division of Pediatric Endocrinology, Cohen Children's Medical
Center of New York/Long Island Jewish Medical Center,
1991 Marcus Avenue, Suite M100, Lake Success, NY 11042, USA

P. Kreitzer, M.D. (✉)
Division of Pediatric Endocrinology, Cohen Children's Medical Center of
New York/Long Island Jewish Medical Center, Lake Success, NY, USA

Hofstra Northwell School of Medicine, Hempstead, NY, USA
e-mail: pkreitzer@nshs.edu

© Springer International Publishing Switzerland 2016
H.L. Appelbaum (ed.), *Abnormal Female Puberty*,
DOI 10.1007/978-3-319-27225-2_5

HCG   Human chorionic gonadotropin
IVF   In vitro fertilization
LH   Luteinizing hormone
MRI   Magnetic resonance imaging
OCP   Oral contraceptive pill
POF   Primary ovarian failure
POI   Primary ovarian insufficiency
PRL   Prolactin
TBG   Thyroid-binding globulin
TSH   Thyroid stimulating hormone
T4   Thyroxine
TS   Turner syndrome

Introduction

Abnormal puberty is a common presenting complaint for pediatric endocrinology and gynecology practices. In girls, normal puberty may begin as early as 8 years [1]. Though most Caucasian females develop breast tissue after the age of 8 years, race plays a role in pubertal timing, as it is more common for African American and Mexican-American females to begin puberty at an earlier age [2]. Activation of the hypothalamic pituitary ovarian axis marks the beginning of puberty. Puberty is initiated in the hypothalamus by an increase in GnRH pulsatility and the subsequent development of the neuroendocrine system allows for changes in gonadal hormone stimulatory and inhibitory effects [3]. Gonadotropins secreted by the pituitary in response to GnRH rise gradually [2]. In early puberty, LH increases at night during sleep but it loses its diurnal pattern near menarche [2]. These hormonal changes of the hypothalamus and pituitary influence the ovary, allowing estrogen levels to gradually rise to adult ranges [3]. Rising estrogen levels account for the development of secondary sexual characteristics and ultimately stimulate endometrial growth allowing for menarche to occur [2].

The Tanner staging method or the Sexual Maturation Rating is commonly used to help standardize pubertal assessment [4]. A prepubertal exam is defined by stage 1 and an adult exam by stage 5

[4, 5]. Most often, the first sign of puberty will be breast or axillary and pubic hair development. A female typically begins breast budding, or thelarche, between the ages of 8–13 years old, with the average age around 10 years [2, 5]. Thelarche and pubarche are followed by a growth spurt and then menarche ensues as the last stage of pubertal development. Menarche is usually achieved 2.5 years after the onset of puberty [5] and puberty is usually completed 2.5–3 years after thelarche begins [6]. Puberty is considered abnormal in a female if the onset is not seen by the age of 13 years or menarche is not achieved by 15 years [6]. Furthermore, menarche is considered delayed if it does not occur within 3 years after pubertal onset [2].

When patients are referred to a specialist due to concerns regarding pubertal delay, the history and physical examination can direct the evaluation. Though the most common cause of delayed puberty is constitutional delay of growth and puberty, which is the diagnosis in 30 % of females with delayed puberty [4, 6], hormonal, genetic and structural causes must be considered. The evaluation and treatment of various hormonal causes of abnormal puberty will be discussed.

Primary Ovarian Insufficiency

Case Presentation

A 14 year old female is referred for evaluation of delayed menarche. She had onset of breast development around 10 years of age, and then gradually progressed through puberty. Four years has passed since the onset of puberty and she has not yet experienced menarche. Her overall health was good, but she complained of experiencing temperature instability over the past 3 weeks (feeling hot and then cold). She had no history of any medical problems and was not taking any medications. She has a normal diet and activity level. Maternal menarche was at the age of 12. Family history includes a maternal history of Hashimoto's thyroiditis, a maternal second cousin with type 1 diabetes, and a maternal aunt with a mosaic form of Turner syndrome.

On examination, her height was 161.2 cm (63.5 in.; 50th percentile), weight was 59 kg (130.5 lbs; 77th percentile), and BMI was 23 kg/m^2 (82nd percentile). Her vital signs were normal. She had no dysmorphic features, hirsutism, or acne. Pubertal status was Tanner 4 breast tissue and Tanner 5 pubic hair distribution. There was no clitoral enlargement, and the urethra, perineum, and anus were normal. Her exam was significant for diffuse enlargement of her thyroid gland, with no palpable nodules.

Laboratory testing included a normal prolactin level, negative pregnancy test, markedly elevated FSH and LH levels, and an immeasurable estradiol level. Her FSH was 120 IU/mL (upper normal limit luteal phase 11.2 µIU/mL), LH was 68.3 IU/mL (upper normal limit luteal phase 11IU/mL), and Estradiol level was <2.5 pg/mL (lower normal limit for a Tanner 4 female is 21 pg/mL; patient's value was in Tanner 1 range). In addition, she was found to have a mildly elevated TSH of 5.82 µIU/mL (upper limit is 4.8 µIU/mL) and a positive thyroid peroxidase antibody of 1120 IU/mL (normal is <34 IU/mL). Her Total T4 was normal and thyroglobulin antibody was negative. A pelvic ultrasound was performed and found to be normal. The uterus measured $5.3 \times 2.2 \times 4.3$ cm, the endometrial lining was 3 mm, the right ovary measured $2.0 \times 0.7 \times 1.2$ cm, and the left ovary measured $3.2 \times 1.4 \times 1.3$ cm.

Repeat testing was performed which confirmed the diagnosis of primary ovarian insufficiency (POI). Further testing was later sent that was negative for ovarian antibodies and antiadrenal antibodies. The patient also had a normal female karyotype (46, XX) and negative analysis for Fragile X premutations.

Discussion

The patient is an adolescent female who has progressed normally through puberty, but has not achieved menarche. Investigation was warranted given that 4 years have elapsed since the onset of pubertal development. When evaluating primary amenorrhea, it is important to first assess the breast tissue and pubic hair, as this can help direct the evaluation. Lack of breast tissue suggests that there has been absence of gonadal function [7]. While our patient has progressed through puberty, she has not achieved menarche, indicating there has been some gonadal function. Physical exam and/or pelvic ultrasound is important to rule out a vaginal or uterine abnormality, as about 15 % of patients with primary amenorrhea have a structural abnormality [7]. Ultrasound can also help differentiate between a pubertal and prepubertal appearance to the internal reproductive organs. A prepubertal uterus measures 2.5–4 cm in length, is no more than 10 mm thick, and is tubular in shape while a pubertal uterus is 5–8 cm in length, 3 cm in width, 1.5 cm thick, and has a pear shape [8]. Ovarian volume also changes throughout puberty and can be calculated by the prolate ellipsoid formula $(L \times H \times W \times 0.523)$ [9]. The volume is 1.2–2.3 cm^3 in prepubertal girls less than 6 years, 2–4 cm^3 in premenarchal girls, and about 8 cm^3 in postmenarchal girls [8].

If there are no obvious abnormalities on examination, initial blood work should include gonadotropins (LH, FSH), an estradiol level, a prolactin level, a TSH, and a pregnancy test [7]. Abnormal gonadotropins may help identify hyper- or hypogonadotropic hypogonadism, though normal gonadotropins do not rule out ovarian failure if a patient's bone age is prepubertal (less than 11 years) [5]. If gonadotropins are normal, pregnancy, hypothyroidism, Cushing syndrome, hyperprolactinemia, hyperandrogenism, obesity, malnutrition, and psychogenic causes must be considered in the evaluation [5, 6, 10].

Our patient's labs were consistent with the diagnosis of hypergonadotropic hypogonadism, otherwise referred to as POI. In this case, the patient was experiencing vasomotor symptoms which can be suggestive of ovarian failure [11]. Other symptoms of ovarian insufficiency could include vaginal dryness, feelings of dysphoria, and difficulty sleeping [10]. POI, which was previously referred to as primary ovarian failure (POF) [12], is diagnosed in females less than 40 years of age who experience amenorrhea in the presence of elevated gonadotropins and a low estrogen state [13]. The term has changed from POF to POI to more accurately reflect the intermittent and possibly unpredictable nature of ovarian function [12]. Though most patients with POI experience ovarian failure after menarche, about 10 % of patients present with primary amenorrhea [10, 14].

Approximately 1 % of girls are affected by POI and [15] the etiology of this condition remains unknown in about 90 % of cases [6, 14]. The most common known cause of ovarian failure is an X-chromosome defect [5]. The physical exam may identify features of Turner syndrome (TS) which can include, but are not limited to, dysmorphic features, short stature, webbed neck, or lack of or incomplete pubertal development [10, 16]. A karyotype is imperative for an accurate diagnosis, because features of Turner syndrome are not always clearly evident; 10 % of TS patients undergo pubertal progression spontaneously and 5 % even experience menarche [5]. Fragile X premutations account for 2 % of POI cases [14]. Finally, autoimmune oophoritis and other associated autoimmune conditions must be considered. Antiadrenal antibodies are found to be positive in 4 % of patients, while the ovarian antibody test lacks specificity and is often not used [10, 14]. Our patient's strong family history of autoimmunity, her significant goiter, and her positive thyroid antibody increased the suspicion of an autoimmune cause.

Management

The treatment for POI consists not only of hormone replacement therapy, but also includes preventing comorbidities and counseling. Replacement therapy, which comprises estrogen and progesterone, is necessary to achieve and maintain the normal hormone levels of a reproductive female. This is important not only to prevent menopausal symptoms, but to maintain bone health, prevent cardiovascular disease and preserve sexual health. Depending upon when ovarian failure occurs, it may also be necessary to assist in the completion of puberty if pubertal progression was interrupted. If the breasts are not fully developed, lower doses of estrogen replacement must be initiated to allow for pubertal progression. Estrogen is gradually increased to adult or maintenance replacement dosing and then progesterone is added to protect the endometrium from long-term complications associated with unopposed estrogen. Pubertal induction is initiated with estrogen treatment alone followed by the sequential addition of progesterone. Progesterone is added sequentially, rather than concomitantly, in order to allow for estrogen to independently stimulate normal breast development because early progesterone exposure to the breast tissue can result in tubular breast formation [12].

Recommended maintenance hormone replacement is 100 µg of estradiol per day plus a 10–12 day course of progesterone monthly [10]. Estradiol can be administered via many routes, such as transdermal, oral, or transvaginal. Transdermal estrogen replacement is preferred due to its avoidance of first-pass effect on the liver [12], which can increase a patient's risk of thromboembolism [17]. Monthly progesterone courses are needed to shed the endometrial lining and thus avoid endometrial hyperplasia/cancer, particularly adenocarcinoma [18]. Oral contraceptives (OCPs) are not the preferred first-line therapy given their higher estrogen content when compared to estrogen patches [10]. While OCPs do prevent pregnancy and decrease the risk of ovarian/endometrial cancer, they can slightly increase a patient's risk of cardiovascular disease [19, 20]. Caution should be used when prescribing these medications if a patient has any risk factors for hypertension, hyperlipidemia, peripheral artery disease, and venous thromboembolism, or they are smokers [20].

In addition to reestablishing physiologic hormonal levels, bone and cardiovascular health must be maintained. Calcium and vitamin D supplements should be administered to help maintain bone integrity. Though there are currently no specific guidelines, it is recommended that a DEXA scan be obtained at diagnosis to assess baseline bone mineral density [10]. In pediatrics, a calculated z score is used to interpret DEXA scan results, as opposed to a t score which is used for adult scans; a z score below negative two (-2) is considered low [21]. Patients should be encouraged to exercise regularly, making sure to include weight-bearing exercises [10] as these types of exercise are known to increase bone mineral density [22].

Additional emphasis should also be placed on providing emotional support. Many reports have documented that most women with the diagnosis of POI experience significant emotional distress [12, 14, 23], with one study documenting that 89 % of girls experienced moderate to severe levels of emotional distress at diagnosis and 84 % experiencing that level of emotional suffering [15]. Though most of these women are unable to conceive naturally, about 5–10 % of patients do conceive spontaneously [12, 14]; therefore, patients must still be counseled on the need for contraception if not intending to become pregnant. Most women are distressed at diagnosis upon learning of their high likelihood of infertility; it is therefore important to discuss potential fertility options through the use of assisted reproductive technology (ART). Ovulation induction agents are often not successful and therefore rarely used, while in vitro fertilization (IVF) using ovum donation often leads to successful pregnancies [24]. Anti-Mullerian hormone levels have been used to measure ovarian reserve in patients with POI to determine if a patient will respond to treatment with an ovulation induction agent [25].

Outcome

The patient was placed on estradiol and progesterone replacement therapy. She was started on an estradiol transdermal patch that provided 0.1 mg/24 h. To initiate a monthly withdrawal bleed, she was also prescribed micronized progesterone 200 mg PO daily for 10 days at the end of each month. DEXA scan was performed 6 months after diagnosis and found to be normal, with a z score of −0.4 SD. Due to the patient's mildly elevated TSH and significant goiter, levothyroxine 88 μg daily was prescribed as well. Future fertility potential was discussed with the parents.

Clinical Pearls/Pitfalls

1. POI must be considered when a patient presents with delayed puberty.
2. A karyotype, analysis for Fragile X premutations, and antiadrenal antibodies may be informative when a patient is diagnosed with POI, although most etiologies of POI remain unclear.

3. POI requires hormonal replacement therapy, consisting of combined estrogen and progesterone replacement.
4. In addition to hormonal replacement, bone, cardiovascular, sexual, and psychological health must be considered.

Hypothyroidism

Case Presentation

A 17-year-old female is referred for evaluation of irregular menses. Pubertal onset was delayed with initiation of breast development at 14 years of age. She had her first and only period at just over 16 years of age. There are no other current complaints. She has a history of systemic lupus erythematosus (SLE) and is currently treated with Plaquenil, Prednisone, and a baby aspirin. She has a normal diet and activity level. There is a family history of SLE, but no other significant medical conditions. Maternal menarche was at age 11.

On examination, her height was 157 cm (61.8 in.), weight was 51.4 kg (113 lbs), and BMI was 20.9 kg/m². Vital signs were all normal and there was no hirsutism or acne. Pubertal status was Tanner 5 for breast tissue and pubic hair distribution. There was no clitoral enlargement and the urethra, perineum, and anus were normal. It was noted on exam that her thyroid gland was diffusely enlarged, with no palpable nodules.

Laboratory results showed normal FSH, LH, Estradiol, 17-hydroxy progesterone, testosterone, DHEAS, and prolactin levels. Serum pregnancy test was negative. Thyroid studies were significant for an elevated TSH of 541 µIU/mL (upper normal limit 4.8 µIU/mL), low Total T4 of 4.4 µg/dL (lower normal limit 4.6 µg/dL), and positive thyroglobulin antibody of 196 IU/mL (normal <40 IU/mL). Thyroid peroxidase antibody was negative. Given her abnormal thyroid function in the presence of a positive thyroid antibody, the patient was diagnosed with Hashimoto's thyroiditis, or autoimmune hypothyroidism.

Discussion

Hypothyroidism is a condition in which the body is unable to produce adequate levels of thyroid hormone [26, 27]. This may be due to primary thyroid disease such as autoimmune thyroid disease (Hashimoto's thyroiditis), inflammation, medication, surgery, radiation, or congenital hypothyroidism; more rarely this may be due to TSH deficiency, or central hypothyroidism [28]. Thyroid hormone is necessary for growth, development, metabolism, and many other physiologic functions [29]. Abnormalities in pubertal development have often been linked to thyroid conditions.

Both delayed puberty and precocious puberty have been documented in patients with hypothyroidism, most commonly due to Hashimoto's thyroiditis [30]. Hypothyroidism more commonly causes delayed puberty, due to delayed growth and maturation [31, 32]. Precocious puberty, though rarely due to hypothyroidism, is thought to be due to the "hormonal overlap syndrome," a spillover effect of TSH on FSH and LH receptors [31, 32]. TSH, LH, FSH, and PRL are thought to have the potential for overlapping actions, as they are all glycoproteins with a common alpha subunit [33]. The exact mechanism for why hypothyroidism causes pubertal abnormalities is unclear, but Dijkstra et al. previously showed in a rat model that an induced hypothyroid state negatively affects folliculogenesis by affecting granulosa cell differentiation [34]. In addition, in both hypo- and hyperthyroidism, alterations in the metabolism of sex steroids and changes in gonadotropin secretion have been noted [35].

Additional menstrual irregularities have been linked to both overactive and underactive thyroid conditions, including amenorrhea, oligomenorrhea, hypomenorrhea, hypermenorrhea, polymenorrhea, and menorrhagia [31, 35, 36]. Thyroid conditions are more likely to cause amenorrhea, but can alternatively cause menorrhagia as a result of anovulatory dysfunctional bleeding [37]. Though described commonly in the past, more recent studies suggest a decreased frequency in the relationship between menstrual disturbances and thyroid conditions, which is most likely due to subclinical thyroid abnormalities being diagnosed and treated earlier than in the past and thus preventing the development of an overtly hypo- or hyperthyroid state [31, 35].

Management

Thyroid replacement is imperative for all patients with overt hypothyroidism and in patients with subclinical hypothyroidism (elevated TSH with normal total and free T4) in whom the TSH is over 10 μIU/mL or have pubertal/menstrual disturbances felt to be due to thyroid dysfunction [26, 38]. Levothyroxine is the standard treatment of choice for hypothyroidism [27] [26].

Outcome

The patient was started on levothyroxine 50 μg once daily for 2 weeks which was then increased to 100 μg daily. One week after starting the medication, menses returned.

Clinical Pearls/Pitfalls

1. Hypothyroidism should be considered in girls presenting with delayed puberty.
2. Hypothyroidism is diagnosed based on an elevated TSH level, except when central hypothyroidism is suspected.
3. Levothyroxine is the recommended treatment for hypothyroidism.
4. When treatment for profound hypothyroidism is initiated, treatment should be started at a lower dose and then titrated in order to prevent complications including dysfunctional bleeding and other menstrual irregularities.
5. In rare cases, hypothyroidism can cause precocious puberty.

Panhypopituitarism

Case Presentation

A 14 year old female is referred to pediatric endocrinology for delayed puberty. She has not had any breast or pubic hair development, and denies vaginal bleeding. She has never had acne, and does not need deodorant. She has no medical problems, and she does not take any medications, vitamins, or supplements. She has a well-balanced diet, but does not exercise regularly. Maternal menarche was at age 10.

On exam, the patient is 156 cm (61.4 in., 10th–25th percentile), and 63 kg (138.6 lb, 75th–90th percentile). Her BMI is 25.8 kg/m² (90th–95th percentile). Her blood pressure is 100/70, which is normal for age. She has multiple nevi on her upper torso. Her breasts are Tanner 1, as is her pubic hair distribution. Her vaginal mucosal membranes are pink and unestrogenized in appearance.

Laboratory evaluation included a TSH and T4, FSH, LH, estradiol, prolactin, DHEAS, CMP, bone age X-ray, and pelvic ultrasound. TSH is in normal range at 4.1 μIU/mL, with a low total T4 of 3.6 μg/dL. FSH is 0.3 mIU/mL, LH is 0.15 mIU/mL, both prepubertal levels, and estradiol and DHEAS levels are unmeasurably low. Her prolactin level is normal at 12.6 ng/mL. The patient's bone age is interpreted as 13–13.5 years old, 1 year delayed from her chronologic age. Pelvic ultrasound revealed small ovaries and a prepubertal uterus.

The patient returns for additional blood work. She has a low cortisol of 1.9 μg/dL and a low free T4 of 0.5 μg/dL. ACTH is also low at 10 pg/mL. Due to the low FSH and LH, the patient has a GnRH stimulation test. Both the FSH and LH do not increase upon administration of GnRH.

This patient had a MRI of her brain to evaluate the structure of her pituitary gland. She was found to have an ectopic posterior pituitary gland and anterior pituitary hypoplasia.

Discussion

There is no evidence of breast development, indicating that the patient has not entered puberty. She also does not have any sign of adrenarche (pubic or axillary hair, or adult body odor). In females, puberty is considered delayed if the patient has not had breast development by 13 years old, or has not had menarche by 15 years old [6] or 3 years after thelarche [39].

Patients with low FSH, LH, and estradiol have hypogonadotrophic hypogonadism. FSH and LH are gonadotropes, produced by the pituitary gland, necessary for the initiation of progression of puberty [40]. This patient's low estradiol level is therefore due to lack of gonadotropin stimulation of the ovaries. The patient also has a low T4, with an inappropriately low TSH. Central hypothyroidism is caused by decreased production of TSH from the pituitary gland, resulting in decreased thyroid hormone production [41].

This patient has exhibited multiple hormone deficiencies. She has low TSH, FSH, LH, and ACTH. These hormones are all produced in the anterior pituitary gland, along with growth hormone and prolactin. Growth hormone is responsible for linear growth and soft tissue growth, and prolactin is mainly responsible for lactation after parturition. Multiple pituitary hormone deficiencies resulting from panhypopituitarism may be caused by tumors, pituitary surgery and radiation, trauma, infection, and genetic defects [42]. In this patient's case, the panhypopituitarism is the result of a congenital hypoplastic anterior pituitary gland identified on MRI.

Management

Treatment of panhypopituitarism involves replacing the patient's deficient hormones. Cortisol is the most critical hormone to replace. Without pituitary ACTH stimulation, the adrenal glands cannot synthesize and release cortisol resulting in secondary adrenal insufficiency.[43] Cortisol deficiency can cause hypoglycemia, hypotension, fatigue, and fever [44]. Patients with any type of adrenal insufficiency require replacement hydrocortisone. People with functioning pituitary and adrenal glands naturally secrete increased cortisol in times of illness and stress [45]. Therefore, when people with adrenal insufficiency are exposed to any physiologic stress, they must increase their hydrocortisone dose. Aside from cortisol, thyroid replacement is essential to regulate metabolism, and is critical for early brain development and growth in young children [44]. Additionally, growth hormone must be replaced [45].

Gonadarche begins when the hypothalamus begins to release GnRH. In turn, GnRH triggers FSH and LH secretion from the pituitary [40]. FSH stimulates the growth of immature ovarian follicles, which secrete estrogens and progesterones. Estradiol is responsible for the development of female sexual characteristics including breast development and changing distribution of body fat. The vaginal mucosa becomes cornified, and the pH of the vagina becomes more acidic [5]. Estrogen is further responsible for bone maturation and epiphyseal fusion [46]. As puberty progresses, GnRH increases in spurts, causing LH and FSH continue to rise in spikes. Estrogen and progesterone stimulate the pituitary to secrete larger quantities of LH and FSH in response to GnRH. This positive feedback leads to the mid-cycle LH surge which triggers a first ovulation [5]. Patients with panhypopituitarism require sex steroid replacement in order to initiate or potentiate pubertal development.

To induce puberty, the patient will first receive low-dose estrogen, which can be given orally or transdermally. The dose is increased slowly over 2 years. This allows the patient to undergo the physical changes of puberty, including breast development. The slow increase of estradiol will also provide the opportunity for continued vertical growth. After about 12–24 months of unopposed estrogen, or if a patient experiences vaginal bleeding, she is given progesterone in cycles [47]. If the progesterone is given too early, it may result in breast deformity, but it must be started once the patient develops a uterine lining to prevent endometrial hyperplasia [40].

Outcome

The patient was started on replacement hydrocortisone, conjugated estrogen 0.3 mg per day, and levothyroxine 75 μg per day. Her estrogen dose was doubled after 1 year, and shortly after this, she was started on medroxyprogesterone for a 10 day course each month. After this, the patient had her first period. Hormone replacement therapy was maintained.

Clinical Pearls/Pitfalls

1. Females with low FSH, LH, and estradiol have hypogonadotropic hypogonadism.
2. If a patient has one or more pituitary hormone deficiencies, panhypopituitarism should be considered.
3. When a girl has hypogonadotropic hypogonadism, puberty should be initiated with incremental doses of estradiol, with subsequent introduction of progesterone to prevent endometrial hyperplasia.
4. Once she has satisfactory breast development, she should receive progesterone to protect the endometrial lining from becoming hyperplastic.

Hyperprolactinemia

Case Presentation

A 16 year old female is referred to pediatric endocrinology for menstrual irregularity. She had menarche at age 14 years old, and experienced normal regular periods for 2 years. However, for the last year, she has only had two periods, most recently 4 months prior to her visit. She also complains of occasional headaches that self-resolve. Her only medical problem is seasonal allergies, for which she takes cetirizine as needed. She denies headaches, vision deficits, or nipple discharge. She has a well-balanced diet, and exercises once a week.

On exam, the patient is 176.5 cm (98th percentile) and 90.6 kg (98th percentile). Her BMI is 29 kg/m^2 (94th percentile). She has mild hirsutism on her upper lip, back, and abdomen. Her breast development is Tanner 5, and her pubic hair distribution is Tanner 5. Her vision exam reveals no gross visual field deficits. Her neurological exam was grossly normal.

Thyroid function tests, electrolytes, and CBC are normal. She had a normal postpubertal LH level of 4.5 mIU/mL, and a normal postpubertal FSH level of 5.2 mIU/mL. However, her estradiol level is unmeasurable at less than 10 pg/mL. Her total testosterone level is normal at 20.7 ng/dL, as is her androstenedione at 127 ng/dL. Prolactin is markedly elevated at 67.4 ng/mL (normal range is 3–24 in females), with an unmeasurable macroprolactin. Beta-HCG is negative. The patient has an MRI of her brain that revealed a subcentimeter midline pituitary microadenoma, without mass effect on the optic nerves.

Discussion

Prolactin is one of six anterior pituitary hormones, and is chiefly responsible for milk production after parturition. It is produced and secreted by the lactotroph cells. Elevated prolactin levels inhibit the pulsatile secretion of GnRH from the hypothalamus, which is required for FSH and LH secretion from the pituitary gland. This lack of FSH and LH results in amenorrhea. Elevated prolactin can also cause a woman to experience galactorrhea. Similarly, the physiologically elevated prolactin level in pregnant and nursing women is partially responsible for the amenorrhea after parturition [48].

Pathologically increased prolactin levels can be caused by lacto-troph adenomas of the pituitary, as is the case in this patient. Pituitary adenomas (prolactinomas) are caused by a monoclonal expansion of single cells in the pituitary, and hormone output depends on the cell type [49]. Large prolactinomas can cause patients to have headaches and visual changes due to mass effect on the optic nerve [48]. Younger patients with prolactinomas can also present with growth failure and pubertal delay. This can result in primary amenorrhea [50]. Craniopharyngiomas are brain tumors derived from primitive pituitary gland tissue that can also produce excess prolactin [51]. Decreased levels of dopamine can cause hyperprolactinemia, as dopamine normally inhibits prolactin release. Medications that commonly lower dopamine include antipsychotic drugs and gastric motility drugs. Specific antihypertensive drugs that lower dopamine include verapamil and methyldopa [52]. Hyperprolactinemia is also seen in patients with untreated primary hypothyroidism, possibly due to increased secretion of TRH from the hypothalamus [53].

Management

Cabergoline is a dopamine D2 receptor agonist. Like dopamine, cabergoline stimulates dopamine receptors, and therefore inhibits prolactin secretion. It reduces the need for patients with prolactinomas to undergo surgical resection, which can result in panhypopituitarism and diabetes insipidus. Side effects of cabergoline include nausea, sleep disturbances, and psychiatric complaints. Bromocriptine, another D2 receptor agonist, has increased side effects, and is less effective than cabergoline [54]. In a comparative study published in 1994, 31 % of women with hyperprolactinemic amenorrhea experienced nausea on cabergoline, compared to 50 % of the women on bromocriptine ($p < 0.001$) [55]. Twelve percent of women discontinued bromocriptine due to intolerance, compared to 3 % of women taking cabergoline ($p < 0.001$) [55]. Patients typically resume menstruation about 8 weeks after starting dopamine agonists [55]. Complete clinical efficacy, defined as two consecutive menses with evidence of ovulation, was seen in 52 % of women on bromocriptine and 72 % of women on cabergoline [55]. However, bromocriptine is the dopamine agonist of choice when a woman is trying to conceive. Both cabergoline and bromocriptine cross the placenta, but women who took cabergoline during their pregnancy have had children with epilepsy and pervasive development disorders [56]. Bromocriptine should be initiated while trying to conceive in order to promote ovulation, and then discontinued when pregnancy is confirmed [56]. Transsphenoidal surgery remains an option for patients who have macroadenomas, or do not improve with dopamine agonists or cannot tolerate their side effects. The patients who undergo surgery have a higher risk of diabetes insipidus and panhypopituitarism, and also have a higher rate of recurrence of the hyperprolactinemia than patients on medical therapy [57].

Outcome

The patient was started on cabergoline therapy. Repeat prolactin level following 2 months of dopamine agonist was normal at 9.3 ng/mL. She began to menstruate regularly each month afterward.

Clinical Pearls/Pitfalls

1. Prolactin is one of six hormones produced and secreted by the anterior pituitary.
2. Prolactin normally rises during pregnancy and lactation.
3. Hyperprolactinemia may result from pituitary adenomas, craniopharyngiomas, medications, or untreated primary hypothyroidism.
4. Dopamine receptor agonists are the appropriate first-line treatment for prolactinomas.

References

1. Nakamoto JM. Myths and variations in normal pubertal development. Western J Med. 2000;172:182–5.
2. Bordini B, Rosenfield R. Normal pubertal development: Part I: the endocrine basis of puberty. Pediatr Rev. 2011;32:223–9.
3. Stang J, Story M. Understanding adolescent eating behaviors. In: Stang J, Story M, editors. Guidelines for adolescent nutrition services. Minneapolis, MN: University of Minnesota School of Public Health; 2005. p. 1–8.
4. Bordini B, Rosenfield R. Normal pubertal development: Part II: clinical aspects of puberty. Pediatr Rev. 2011;37:281–91.
5. Rosenfield R, Cooke D, Radovick S. The ovary and female maturation. In: Sperling M, editor. Pediatric endocrinology. 3rd ed. Pittsburgh: Saunders; 2008. p. 564–78.
6. Dwyer A, Phan-Hug F, Hauschild M, Elowe-Gruau E, Pitteloud N. Hypogonadism in adolescence. Eur J Endocrinol. 2015;173(1):R15–24.
7. Medicine TPCotASfR. Current evaluation of amenorrhea. Fertil Steril. 2008;90:S219–S25.
8. Garel L, Dubois J, Grignon A, Filiatrault D, Vliet GV. US of the pediatric female pelvis: a clinical perspective. Radiographics. 2001;21:1393–407.
9. Pavlik EJ, DePriest PD, Gallion HH, et al. Ovarian volume related to age. Gynecol Oncol. 2000;77:410–2.
10. Nelson L. Primary ovarian insufficiency. New Engl J Med. 2009;360:606–14.
11. Menopause. American Congress of Obstetricians and Gynecologists, 2013. Accessed February 26, 2015, at http://www.acog.org/Patients/FAQs/Menopause.
12. American Congress of Obstetricians and Gynecologists. Primary ovarian insufficiency in adolescents and young women. 2014. Accessed February

26, 2015, at http://www.acog.org/%20Resources-And-Publications/ Committee-Opinions/Committee-on-Adolescent-Health-Care/ Primary-Ovarian-Insufficiency-in-Adolescents-and-Young-Women.

13. Carr BR. Disorders of the ovaries and female reproductive tract. In: Wilson JD et al., editors. William's textbook of endocrinology. 9th ed. Philadelphia: W.B. Saunders; 1998. p. 485.

14. Rafique S, Sterling E, Nelson L. A new approach to primary ovarian insufficiency. Obstet Gynecol Clin North Am. 2012;39:567–86.

15. Groff A, Covington S, Halverson L, et al. Assessing the emotional needs of women with spontaneous premature ovarian failure. Fertil Steril. 2005;83:1734–41.

16. Gravholt C. Epidemiological, endocrine and metabolic features in Turner syndrome. Eur J Endocrinol. 2004;151:657–87.

17. Simon J. What's new in hormone replacement therapy: Focus on transdermal estradiol and micronized progesterone. Climacteric. 2012;15:3–10.

18. Lignières B. Oral micronized progesterone. Clin Ther. 1999;21:41–60.

19. Sherif K. Benefits and risks of oral contraceptives. Am J Obstet Gynecol. 1999;180:S343–S8.

20. Fehr AD, Mounsey A, Yates JE, Flake D. Cardiovascular risks of combined oral contraceptive use. Am Fam Physician. 2012;86:1–2.

21. Pediatrics AAo. Bone densitometry in children and adolescents. Pediatrics. 2011;127:189–94.

22. Etherington J, Harris PA, Nandra D, et al. The effect of weight-bearing exercise on bone mineral density: a study of female ex-elite athletes and the general population. J Bone Miner Res. 1996;11:1333–8.

23. Eunice Kennedy Shriver National Institute of Child Health and Human Development. What are the treatments for POI? 2013. Accessed February 26, 2015, at https://www.nichd.nih.gov/health/topics/poi/conditioninfo/Pages/treatments.aspx.

24. Shelling AN. Premature ovarian failure. Reproduction. 2010;140:633–41.

25. Bidet M, Bachelot A, Touraine P. Premature ovarian failure: predictability of intermittent function and response to ovulation induction agents. Curr Opin Obstet Gynecol. 2008;20:416–20.

26. Khandelwal D, Tandon N. Overt and subclinical hypothyroidism: who to treat and how. Drugs. 2012;72:17–33.

27. Almandoz J, Gharib H. Hypothyroidism: etiology, diagnosis, and management. Med Clin North Am. 2012;96:203–21.

28. National Institute of Diabetes and Digestive and Kidney Disorders. Hypothyroidism. 2013. Accessed February 26, 2015, at http://www.niddk.nih.gov/health-information/health-topics/endocrine/hypothyroidism/Pages/fact-sheet.aspx.

29. Yen PM. Physiological and molecular basis of thyroid hormone action. Physiol Rev. 2001;81:1097–142.

30. Weber G, Vigone M, Chiumello G. Thyroid function and puberty. J Pediatr Endocrinol Metab. 2003;16:S253–7.

31. Koutras D. Disturbances of menstruation in thyroid disease. Ann N Y Acad Sci. 1997;816:280–4.
32. Indumathi C, Bantwal G, Patil M. Primary hypothyroidism with precocious puberty and bilateral cystic ovaries. Indian J Pediatr. 2007;74:781–3.
33. Dijkstra G, de Rooij DG, de Jong FH, van den Hurk R. Effect of hypothyroidism on ovarian follicular development, granulosa cell proliferation and peripheral hormone levels in the prepubertal rat. Eur J Endocrinol. 1996;134:649–54.
34. Krassas GE. Thyroid disease and female reproduction. Fertil Steril. 2000;74:1063–70.
35. Kakuno Y, Amino N, Kanoh M, Kawai M, Fujiwara M. Menstrual disturbances in various thyroid diseases. Endocr J. 2010;57:1017–22.
36. Krassas G, Pontikides N, Kaltsas T, et al. Disturbances of menstruation in hypothyroidism. Clin Endocrinol (Oxf). 1999;50:655–9.
37. Livingstone M, Fraser IS. Mechanisms of abnormal uterine bleeding. Hum Reprod Update. 2002;8:60–7.
38. Kaplowitz P. Subclinical hypothyroidism in children: normal variation or sign of a failing thyroid gland? Int J Pediatr Endocrinol. 2010;2010:281453.
39. Medicine PCotASfR. Current evaluation of amenorrhea. Fertil Steril. 2006;86:S148.
40. Viswanathan V, Eugster E. Etiology and treatment of hypogonadism in adolescents. Pediatr Clin North Am. 2011;58:1181–200.
41. Samuels MH, Ridgway EC. Central hypothyroidism. Endocrinol Metab Clin North Am. 1992;21:903–19.
42. Prabhakar V, Shalet S. Aetiology, diagnosis, and management of hypopituitarism in adult life. Postgrad Med J. 2006;82:259–66.
43. Grossman AB. The diagnosis and management of central hypoadrenalism. J Clin Endocrinol Metabol. 2010;95:4855–63.
44. Mullur R, Liu Y-Y, Brent GA. Thyroid hormone regulation of metabolism. Physiol Rev. 2014;94:355–82.
45. Ross J, Czernichow P, Biller BMK, Colao A, Reiter E, Kiess W. Growth hormone: health considerations beyond height gain. Pediatrics. 2010;125:e906–18.
46. Emons J, Chagin AS, Sävendahl L, Karperien M, Wit JM. Mechanisms of growth plate maturation and epiphyseal fusion. Horm Res Paediatr. 2011;75:383–91.
47. DiVasta A, Gordon C. Hormone replacement therapy and the adolescent. Curr Opin Obstet Gynecol. 2010;22:363–8.
48. Mancini T, Casanueva FF, Giustina A. Hyperprolactinemia and prolactinomas. Endocrinol Metab Clin North Am. 2008;37:67–99.
49. Herman V et al. Clonal origin of pituitary adenomas. J Clin Endocrinol Metabol. 1990;71:1427–33.
50. Saranac L, Zivanovic S, Radovanovic Z, Kostic G, Markovic I. Hyperprolactinemia: different clinical expression in childhood. Horm Res Paediatr. 2010;73:187–92.

51. Halac I, Zimmerman D. Endocrine manifestations of craniopharyngioma. Childs Nerv Syst. 2005;21:640–8.
52. Molitch ME. Drugs and prolactin. Pituitary. 2008;11:209–18.
53. Snyder PJ, Jacobs LS, Utiger RD, Daughaday WH. Thyroid hormone inhibition of the prolactin response to thyrotropin-releasing hormone. J Clin Invest. 1973;52:2324–9.
54. Wang AT et al. Treatment of hyperprolactinemia: a systemic review and meta-analysis. Syst Rev. 2012;1:33.
55. Webster J, Piscitelli G, Polli A, Ferrari CI, Ismail I, Scanlon MF. A comparison of cabergoline and bromocriptine in the treatment of hyperprolactinemic amenorrhea. N Engl J Med. 1994;331:904–9.
56. Shibli-Rahhal A, Schlecte J. Hyperprolactinemia and infertility. Endocrinol Metab Clin North Am. 2011;40:837–46.
57. Melmed S, Kleinberg D. Pituitary masses and tumors. In: Melmed S, Polonsky K, Larsen R, Kronenberg H, editors. Williams textbook of endocrinology. 12th ed. Philadelphia: Elsevier Saunders; 2011. p. 229–90.

Chapter 6
Androgenic Disorders and Abnormal Pubertal Development

Phyllis W. Speiser

Abbreviations

17OHP	17-Hydroxyprogesterone
BMI	Body mass index
CNS	Central nervous system
DOC	Deoxycorticosterone
GC	Glucocorticoid
MAS	McCune–Albright syndrome
MCR	Mineralocorticoid receptor
[N]CAH	[Nonclassic] congenital adrenal hyperplasia
PCOS	Polycystic ovarian syndrome

P.W. Speiser, M.D. (✉)
Division of Pediatric Endocrinology, Cohen Children's Medical
Center of NY, 1991 Marcus Ave., Suite M100,
Lake Success, NY 11042, USA

Hofstra Northwell School of Medicine, Hempstead, NY, USA
e-mail: pspeiser@nshs.edu

© Springer International Publishing Switzerland 2016
H.L. Appelbaum (ed.), *Abnormal Female Puberty*,
DOI 10.1007/978-3-319-27225-2_6

Introduction

Symptoms of androgen excess in children and adolescents are a frequent cause for referrals to the endocrinologist or gynecologist. Typical referrals may involve a girl with premature pubarche or a teen with irregular menses, unwanted facial or body hair, and/or acne. History and physical examination provide important clues as to the chronicity, severity, and exact nature of the complaints. The clinician should gather information dating back to birth, including birth weight. Small birth weight and rapid postnatal catch-up growth have been associated with disordered growth and puberty [1], as well as metabolic syndrome and diabetes [2, 3]. Ethnicity, race, and family medical history are similarly important, as there are androgenic disorders that affect distinct population subgroups. In examining the patients, particular attention should be paid to dermatologic manifestations of androgen excess. The location and severity of acne vulgaris should be noted. The Ferriman–Gallwey score can provide a semi-objective description of the location and severity of excess facial and body hair [4]; a score of ≥8 is indicative of clinically significant hirsutism. A description of the location and severity of excess of facial and body hair should be addressed. Laboratory determinations should be done in a laboratory employing a high degree of quality control with reference standards for women's and children's hormone measurements. The key distinctions are whether the androgen profile is within normal limits for gender, age, and Tanner pubertal stage [5]. Additionally, the pattern of androgen or androgen precursors will help discern the source of androgen production: adrenal, ovarian, or tumoral. These results aid in the decision of how to best treat the patient. Imaging studies may be used judiciously to augment these findings, particularly in the case of markedly elevated testosterone levels.

At the other end of the spectrum, and less frequently seen, are conditions in which there is inadequate sex hormone production and delayed or absent pubertal changes. The latter cases may be difficult to distinguish from idiopathic or functional causes of pubertal disruption. A complete evaluation will often require dynamic tests of the pituitary–adrenal or pituitary–ovarian axes, along with a more in-depth search for genetic causes. This chapter will provide a case-based approach to solving typical cases of abnormal androgen metabolism and the resulting abnormal signs of pubertal development.

Case 1: Presentation

A 16-year-old female is referred for irregular periods. She had menarche at 13 years, and was getting periods on average about every 6 months that lasted only 1–2 days. Her last menstrual period was 2 months ago and lasted just 1 day. Her general health is good. She does not exercise excessively and eats a healthy, balanced diet. The only pertinent family history is that two paternal aunts were infertile.

On examination, her height was 147 cm (58 in.) and weight 44.5 kg (98 lbs); BMI was 22. Her blood pressure was normal. General habitus was normal for a young woman. She had no acne or hirsutism. Pubertal status was Tanner stage 5 for breasts and pubic hair; there was no clitoral enlargement.

Laboratory tests included normal thyroid functions, prolactin, luteinizing hormone (LH), follicle-stimulating hormone (FSH), estradiol, sex hormone binding globulin, and DHEA-sulfate (DHEAS). Her early morning 17-hydroxyprogesterone (17OHP; tandem mass spectrometry assay) was markedly elevated at 1800 ng/dL with mildly elevated testosterone of 44 ng/dL (upper normal limit 38) and androstenedione of 310 ng/dL (upper normal limit 240).

Case 1: Discussion

Prominent in the history are very infrequent and scanty menses and the absence of virilizing features. The family history suggests this may be an inherited disorder. The clinical features might be considered typical of the non-ovulatory menstrual pattern of early adolescence, or due to functional hypothalamic oligo- or amenorrhea [6]. However, the patient is already three years past menarche, and should have a more frequent cyclical regular pattern. She does not have a history suggestive of an eating disorder associated with amenorrhea. The lack of hirsutism and acne suggest, if anything, a mild form of androgen excess. It might be tempting to label this young woman as having polycystic ovarian syndrome (PCOS), but it is important to first exclude other causes of oligomenorrhea [7]. Nonclassic congenital adrenal hyperplasia (NCAH), or late-onset congenital adrenal hyperplasia, is prevalent in the general population with up to 1 in 100 individuals affected, with higher prevalence in select inbred ethnic groups, such as Ashkenazi (Eastern European) Jews [8]. NCAH often mimics the phenotype of PCOS; however, these two conditions mandate different forms of treatment.

The patient's lab data are notable for a selectively elevated 17OHP level. Even without cosyntropin (ACTH 1-24) stimulation, a blood sample obtained before 8 am in the early follicular phase (if the patient is regularly cycling) is often diagnostic, as endogenous ACTH peaks between 4 and 8 am causing the early morning rise in adrenal cortical hormone secretion. A 17OHP level of >1000 ng/dL by tandem mass spectrometry is consistent with the nonclassic or mild form of congenital adrenal hyperplasia (NCAH) owing to steroid 21-hydroxylase deficiency [9]. Note that screening serum 17OHP measurements done late in the day are not informative. In cases where the 17OHP is only slightly high at baseline, cosyntropin stimulation is recommended to confirm the diagnosis by measuring a full panel of related adrenal steroids. Note that DHEA-sulfate is not elevated, and the testosterone is only slightly above the upper normal limit for women. Androstenedione, an immediate precursor to testosterone in the steroid synthetic pathway, is also often measurably elevated in NCAH. It is helpful to measure both testosterone and androstenedione, since these levels do not fluctuate as much with time of day as 17OHP. Note that unless one measures 17OHP to make the diagnosis of this disorder of steroid synthesis, other nonspecific laboratory measures will not be informative. Genotyping for CYP21A2 mutations is not essential for making initial treatment decisions in adolescents. However, genetic counseling is recommended for patients interested in pregnancy [9]. As of this writing, the cost of genotyping remains high and should be reserved for situations where the results will affect patient management.

Case 1: Management

The first-line treatment for NCAH in symptomatic individuals is low dose hydrocortisone, generally not more than 10–15 mg/m^2/day in two divided doses. This medication is preferred due to the short half-life and lower potency among this class of steroids, potentially avoiding adverse side effects that accompany treatment with either prednisone of dexamethasone [9]. The goal of therapy is to reduce excessive androgen secretion by replacing a partial deficiency of cortisol characteristic of this inborn error in steroid synthesis. Proper treatment with glucocorticoid (GC) medication will promptly restore adrenal hormone equilibrium and consequently allow resumption of normal ovulation and menstrual cycles, usually within about 3 months [10]. Hirsutism and acne will be ameliorated over a longer time frame. In younger girls detected with advanced bone age, treatment will allow for normal growth and pubertal development. If symptoms do not resolve with glucocorticoid treatment, other ancillary treatments may be considered. Combination estrogen/progestin contraceptive regimens can support regular menses, but do not treat the underlying disorder. If fertility is desired, and glucocorticoids have not achieved this goal, then assisted reproductive technologies may be helpful. It is important to note that pregnancy is achieved spontaneously in most cases, but that there may be subfecundity in the pregnancies achieved without glucocorticoid treatment [10, 11]. Cosmetic hair removal and aggressive dermatologic treatment of severe acne may help self-image.

Serum 17OHP, androstenedione, and testosterone are the best indicators of the adequacy of GC treatment. Normal levels of 17OHP and the other steroids are not a treatment goal, but instead indicate over-treatment [9]. ACTH measurements are not useful for a diagnostic or therapeutic profile. Acceptably treated NCAH patients generally have mildly elevated steroid levels. Once symptoms resolve and fertility is not at issue, one can consider tapering and discontinuing glucocorticoids permanently. Affected individuals should be reassured that NCAH is not a life-threatening condition, and most patients have no clinically significant cortisol deficiency. There is no evidence of any associated endometrial hyperplasia or cancer risk in NCAH patients due to chronic anovulation, nor is it uniformly associated with fertility problems.

Outcome

The young woman was treated with hydrocortisone 5 mg twice daily. Within 1 month, her adrenal hormone levels were adequately suppressed. Menses became regular after 3 months on treatment. She has experienced no adverse side effects of this treatment.

Clinical Pearls/Pitfalls

1. Irregular menses may be caused by hyperandrogenic disorders other than PCOS.
2. An early morning serum 17-hydroxyprogesterone measured by LC/MS/MS may reveal the diagnosis of nonclassic 21-hydroxylase deficiency CAH.
3. Low dose glucocorticoid treatment quickly reverses menstrual irregularity and anovulatory periods in NCAH.

Case 2: Presentation

A 7-year-old girl is referred for early onset of axillary and pubic hair, first noticed about a year earlier. Her height tracked between the 50–60 % over the prior 2 years; weight was 75 %. There was no pertinent prior medical history or family history, and no known exposure to hormones. Her midparent height was at the 50 %.

Physical examination was notable for height and weight at the 65 %. Blood pressure was normal. She had a few facial comedones. Pubertal status was Tanner stage 1 breasts and Tanner stage 3 pubic hair. There was no clitoral enlargement and the external genitalia were normal.

Laboratory tests showed an elevated baseline serum 17OHP of 350 ng/dL, prompting a cosyntropin stimulation test in which her 60 min 17OHP value was elevated at 4490 ng/dL. Testosterone was mildly elevated for a girl of 7 at 13 ng/dL (upper normal 10). Cortisol stimulated normally, and there were no other abnormalities on her comprehensive hormonal profile including cortisol, androstenedione, and DHEAS, among other analytes. There was no evidence of any blood electrolyte, glucose, or liver function abnormalities. Bone age was read as 11 years at chronologic age 9 years 8 months, within 2 SD of chronologic age.

Case 2: Discussion

Guidelines for recognizing precocious pubarche and thelarche have been revised so that children as young as 7 may have Tanner stage 2 pubic hair or breasts, and still be considered normal [12]. This is only true if multiple signs of puberty are absent and there is no growth spurt or advancing bone age. Obese children of all ethnicities and races, and children of African American or Latino background may show pubertal signs earlier than lean Caucasian children [13, 14]. Adrenarche is characterized by indolent body hair development and gradually rising serum DHEA-sulfate [15]. Precocious adrenarche's hallmark is higher than expected DHEA-sulfate, and sometimes androstenedione and testosterone, but not 17OHP [16]. In our case, this non-obese child, pubarche began at 6 and rapidly progressed, seldom a normal finding.

The differential diagnosis for isolated early onset pubic hair, other than idiopathic precocious pubarche/adrenarche, includes exogenous androgen exposure, a tumoral source of androgen, or a mild inborn error of steroid metabolism causing androgen excess. Since many men are now treated with transdermal testosterone, inadvertent exposure of women and children is a real concern [17].

Parents should be questioned about use of non-prescription nutritional and health supplements that may not be FDA-regulated. There has been at least one series of cases involving female virilization following inadvertent exposure to a potent synthetic androgen contaminating vitamin preparations [18]. Additional sources of androgens may include so-called endocrine disruptors from environmental pollutants [19, 20]. In these instances, serum testosterone is often not measurably elevated. Brain tumors, most commonly germ cell tumors secreting HCG, or CNS tumors impinging on the pineal, hypothalamus or pituitary, will often produce rapidly progressive puberty [21]. Sources of non-gonadotropin-dependent precocious puberty include sex cord tumors of the gonads or adrenal carcinomas that directly secrete estrogens, androgens, and in some instances, cortisol or aldosterone. McCune–Albright syndrome (MAS) is a tumor syndrome due to sporadic activating mutations in the GNAS1 gene that cause constitutive activation of sex hormone production and suppressed gonadotropins. MAS should be considered in the setting of café au lait skin lesions, fibrous bone dysplasia, gonadal cysts or hypertrophy, and/or other endocrine gland tumors [22].

The lab results described above confirm an adrenal source of androgen excess consistent with NCAH due to steroid 21-hydroxylase deficiency. This presentation is absolutely typical of this condition in which relative cortisol deficiency results in overproduction of adrenal androgen precursors. As implied by the term "nonclassic," affected children do not suffer all the complications observed with the classic infantile onset disease. Thus, they have normal sodium balance and no genital ambiguity in 46, XX females [8]. The clinician's dilemma is whether to treat individuals with subtle signs of androgen excess with glucocorticoids. The Endocrine Society's Clinical Practice Guidelines based on expert opinion concluded that there is no direct evidence that treatment of minimally symptomatic children or adolescents is necessary [9].

Case 2: Management

In this particular case, the only sign of androgen excess is early pubic hair. There has been no growth acceleration, significant bone age advancement, acne, or hirsutism. Therefore, the prudent approach is to continue to observe this child regularly for any new problems without glucocorticoid treatment. Parents should be informed of potential signs of androgen excess, such as worsening acne, rapid statural growth, or hirsutism in a child that could indicate progression, and should be instructed to call these to medical attention early.

Case 2: Outcome

The child continued to grow normally. Although pubarche was accelerated, all other secondary sexual characteristics developed in a timely manner. Serum measurements of adrenal androgen precursors showed persistently, mildly elevated 17OHP and androstenedione. Glucocorticoid treatment was not recommended.

Case 2: Clinical Pearls

1. Premature pubarche may be due to a nonclassic form of CAH.
2. Glucocorticoid treatment is not always recommended in a child with steady, normal statural growth and gradual progression of puberty.

Case 3: Presentation

A 15-year-old young woman presents with hypertension and primary amenorrhea. The pregnancy and birth history were unremarkable. The parents had been told that the girl had hypertension during a brief hospitalization at age 7, but she was never treated with antihypertensive medications. Her general health is described as excellent, and her patterns of growth and weight gain were entirely normal. The patient denies exposure to any drugs, chemicals, or hormones. Mother experienced menarche at 13, and neither she nor any female relatives had fertility problems or androgen excess. There was a family history of hypertension in both sets of grandparents.

On examination her height is at the 70 %; BMI 83 %. Blood pressure is >95 % at 144/92. She has Tanner 2 breasts; Tanner 1 pubic hair. There is no clitoral enlargement or labial fusion. There is no evidence of acne or hirsutism.

Baseline laboratory tests show low levels of testosterone and estradiol with high gonadotropins. Karyotype is normal female, 46, XX. A transabdominal pelvic ultrasound shows a small uterus and ovaries.

Case 3: Discussion

The salient features distinguishing this from the usual case of delayed puberty or absent menses are the low levels of estrogen with high gonadotropins, and the utter lack of virilizing signs or symptoms. Thus, it is not logical to suspect the more common virilizing types of CAH. The most frequent genetic cause of pubertal delay and amenorrhea is monosomy X (45, X), indicative of Turner Syndrome. This condition found in ~1:2500 births is often associated with hypertension, but in the setting of multiple phenotypic anomalies, e.g., short stature, low set ears, webbed neck, shield chest, renal anomalies, and aortic coarctation [23]. This patient's presentation cannot be attributed to Turner syndrome, since she has two X chromosomes. Alternative causes of premature ovarian failure or insufficiency (POF/POI) must be considered. Galactosemia is an inborn error of metabolism usually diagnosed by newborn screening and treated with a galactose elimination diet. Females who have not had the benefit of galactose restrictive diets tend to develop POI [24]. Fragile X testing, anti-ovarian and anti-21-hydroxylase antibody titers are among the readily available tests recommended to exclude a genetic syndrome or autoimmune acquired diseases causing POF [25]. In our case, there is no history suggesting a high risk for acquired ovarian failure, such as chemotherapeutic agents or radiation exposure. Certainly, none of the aforementioned conditions would adequately explain a phenotypically normal young woman with POF in association with hypertension.

We are so often concerned with hyperandrogenic conditions that disorders associated with lack of sex hormone production can easily be overlooked. The most common form of congenital adrenal hyperplasia (CAH) is steroid 21-hydroxylase deficiency associated with virilization of females, discussed above in reference to the nonclassic forms of this condition. Among the non-virilizing and hypertensive forms of CAH is steroid 17-hydroxylase/17,20 lyase deficiency. This enzyme deficiency interrupts the pathway leading to the C19 steroids that serve as precursors to both testosterone and estrogens [26]. As a consequence, mineralocorticoids accumulate causing sodium retention and hypertension. The hallmarks of mineralocorticoid hypertension are low plasma renin activity and variable hypokalemia. To confirm this diagnosis, it is necessary to perform an ACTH (cosyntropin) stimulation test. This showed elevated baseline and stimulated progesterone and deoxycorticosterone (DOC), precursors to 17-hydroxylase. DOC is a ligand for the mineralocorticoid receptor (MCR), causing hypertension when present in high concentrations. Genotyping CYP17 can provide further confirmation, especially if hormone tests are equivocal.

Case 3: Management

Treatment is aimed at controlling the hypertension first. This is accomplished initially by suppressing ACTH and thereby DOC with low dose glucocorticoid, such as hydrocortisone. Ancillary antihypertensive treatment may be required with a potassium-sparing MCR antagonist such as spironolactone or the more selective MCR antagonist, eplerenone [27, 28]. Once blood pressure is controlled, sex hormone replacement may be initiated. Current expert opinion favors starting with low dose transdermal estrogen delivery, with gradual dose escalation until the full adult dose is reached [29]. Women with CAH due to 17-hydroxylase deficiency are infertile, but may benefit from ovum donation, since the uterus and other internal organs are intact [26].

Case 3: Outcome

This young woman was treated with low dose glucocorticoids and combined estrogen/progestin replacement. Her blood pressure continued to be mildly elevated and she was also treated with antihypertensive medication in the form of an angiotensin II receptor blocker with improved blood pressures.

Case 3: Clinical Pearls

1. The combination of delayed puberty, amenorrhea, and hypertension in a 46, XX individual is highly suggestive of the rare form of CAH due to 17-hydroxylase/17, 20-hydroxylase deficiency.
2. The therapeutic approach to this condition must address suppression of adrenal mineralocorticoids, hormone replacement, and adequate control of hypertension.

Case 4: Presentation

A 15-year-old female presents with amenorrhea and progressively worsening hirsutism requiring facial hair waxing every 2–3 weeks for the past year. Breast development began at age 11 and pubic hair has been present for longer. She does not exercise and she eats a high carbohydrate diet. She has not been treated with any medications to alleviate the symptoms and she does not take vitamins or supplements.

Examination shows BMI in the mildly obese range at the 96 %. She has extensive terminal hair growth on the face and trunk (Ferriman–Gallwey score of 27/44, where >8 is considered hirsute). There is no androgenic pattern hair loss or acne. Pubertal status is Tanner stage 5. There is no clitoral enlargement on inspection of the external genitalia. Laboratory results reveal elevated serum testosterone of 69 ng/dL (upper normal limit 40) and androstenedione 295 ng/dL (upper normal limit 240). LH, FSH, estradiol, DHEAS, and 17OHP were normal. A pelvic ultrasound was unremarkable.

Case 4: Discussion

This patient has severe hirsutism in addition to oligomenorrhea. Her measurably high levels of testosterone and androstenedione and normal levels of 17OHP and DHEAS suggest an ovarian source of hyperandrogenism. Unlike CAH, there is no single diagnostic test that can absolutely confirm the diagnosis of PCOS and ovarian morphology on transabdominal ultrasound is not considered as informative in adolescents as in adult women, mainly because ovarian cysts and irregular menses are commonplace, but transient, in teens [30]. NIH [31] and Androgen Excess-PCOS Society [32] criteria for PCOS include chronic anovulation AND clinical and/or biochemical signs of hyperandrogenism with exclusion of other etiologies, e.g., CAH or ovarian tumors. Treatment of PCOS should be directed at restoring regular menses, alleviating hyperandrogenic symptoms, and prevention of long-term complications associated with chronic anovulation such as endometrial hyperplasia or endometrial cancer. To achieve these goals, The Endocrine Society's Clinical Practice Guidelines for PCOS selected contraceptives as the first treatment of choice [7]. Adding spironolactone has no beneficial effect [33]. Outside the US, cyproterone acetate has been found associated with additive anti-androgenic benefits, specifically, higher sex hormone binding levels and lower Ferriman–Gallwey scores for hirsutism over at least a 1 year period of observation [34]. Drospirenone, a newer progestin found in preparations available in the US, has similar properties [34]. A large systematic review and meta-analysis found no clear evidence that drospirenone increases thromboembolism risk compared to other combined contraceptives [35].

Patients with PCOS are at risk for development of obesity, type 2 diabetes, and metabolic syndrome [36]. Appropriate nutritional and dietary recommendations should be made and regular cardiovascular exercise should be encouraged. Metformin may be considered, especially if the patient is at high risk type 2 diabetes due to high BMI, race or ethnicity, positive family history, presence of acanthosis nigricans, or biochemical evidence of hyperglycemia [7]. Patients should be regularly monitored while on treatment and informed of potential adverse side effects for each drug. It is rare for adolescents to experience the lactic acidosis reported in adults taking Metformin, and elevated liver transaminases are not an absolute contraindication to using this drug [37].

Case 4: Management

The patient was treated with an oral contraceptive in the form of ethinyl estradiol plus drospirenone. Lifestyle changes to include regular cardiovascular exercise and a carbohydrate controlled diet were encouraged.

Case 4: Outcome

Regular menses were promptly restored on combined estrogen/ progestin treatment. Resolution of hirsutism occurred much more slowly. The patient was advised to use concomitant cosmetic hair removal modalities to alleviate these symptoms, and to intensify lifestyle management of excess weight gain. Since she was not considered high risk for type 2 diabetes, metformin was not prescribed.

Case 4: Clinical Pearls

1. The diagnosis of PCOS in teenagers is more complicated than in adult women. Girls within the first 2–5 post-menarchal years may experience irregular menses. Moreover, in the teenage years, multiple follicle cysts are often seen on ultrasound.
2. Management should include hormonal therapy and lifestyle changes such as behavior modification including regular cardio-vascular exercise and carbohydrate controlled diet.

Summary

These cases illustrate the importance of considering disorders of both adrenal and ovaries, both those associated with excessive and inadequate sex hormone production, as potential causes of abnormal puberty. Clearly, the approach to treatment of the various forms of CAH discussed herein warrants specific types of treatment that address the root cause of sex hormone imbalance. Ovarian hyperandrogenism requires different treatment approaches.

References

1. Ibanez L, Lopez-Bermejo A, Diaz M, Marcos MV. Endocrinology and gynecology of girls and women with low birth weight. Fetal Diagn Ther. 2011;30(4):243–9.
2. Barker DJ, Hales CN, Fall CH, Osmond C, Phipps K, Clark PM. Type 2 (non-insulin-dependent) diabetes mellitus, hypertension and hyperlipidaemia (syndrome X): relation to reduced fetal growth. Diabetologia. 1993;36(1):62–7.
3. Beardsall K, Ong KK, Murphy N, Ahmed ML, Zhao JH, Peeters MW, et al. Heritability of childhood weight gain from birth and risk markers for adult metabolic disease in prepubertal twins. J Clin Endocrinol Metab. 2009;94(10):3708–13.
4. Rosenfield RL. Clinical practice. Hirsutism. N Engl J Med. 2005;353(24):2578–88.
5. Rosner W, Vesper H. Toward excellence in testosterone testing: a consensus statement. J Clin Endocrinol Metab. 2010;95(10):4542–8.
6. Gordon CM. Clinical practice. Functional hypothalamic amenorrhea. N Engl J Med. 2010;363(4):365–71.
7. Legro RS, Arslanian SA, Ehrmann DA, Hoeger KM, Murad MH, Pasquali R, et al. Diagnosis and treatment of polycystic ovary syndrome: an Endocrine Society clinical practice guideline. J Clin Endocrinol Metab. 2013;98(12):4565–92.
8. Speiser PW, White PC. Congenital adrenal hyperplasia. N Engl J Med. 2003;349(8):776–88.
9. Speiser PW, Azziz R, Baskin LS, Ghizzoni L, Hensle TW, Merke DP, et al. Congenital adrenal hyperplasia due to steroid 21-hydroxylase deficiency: an Endocrine Society clinical practice guideline. J Clin Endocrinol Metab. 2010;95(9):4133–60.
10. Bidet M, Bellanne-Chantelot C, Galand-Portier MB, Golmard JL, Tardy V, Morel Y, et al. Fertility in women with nonclassical congenital adrenal hyperplasia due to 21-hydroxylase deficiency. J Clin Endocrinol Metab. 2010;95(3):1182–90.
11. Moran C, Azziz R, Weintrob N, Witchel SF, Rohmer V, Dewailly D, et al. Reproductive outcome of women with 21-hydroxylase-deficient nonclassic adrenal hyperplasia. J Clin Endocrinol Metab. 2006;91(9):3451–6.

12. Kaplowitz PB, Oberfield SE. Reexamination of the age limit for defining when puberty is precocious in girls in the United States: implications for evaluation and treatment. Drug and Therapeutics and Executive Committees of the Lawson Wilkins Pediatric Endocrine Society. Pediatrics. 1999;104(4 Pt 1):936–41.

13. Addo OY, Miller BS, Lee PA, Hediger ML, Himes JH. Age at hormonal onset of puberty based on luteinizing hormone, inhibin B, and body composition in preadolescent U.S. girls. Pediatr Res. 2014;76(6):564–70.

14. Corvalan C, Uauy R, Mericq V. Obesity is positively associated with dehydroepiandrosterone sulfate concentrations at 7 y in Chilean children of normal birth weight. Am J Clin Nutr. 2013;97(2):318–25.

15. Palmert MR, Hayden DL, Mansfield MJ, Crigler Jr JF, Crowley Jr WF, Chandler DW, et al. The longitudinal study of adrenal maturation during gonadal suppression: evidence that adrenarche is a gradual process. J Clin Endocrinol Metab. 2001;86(9):4536–42.

16. von Oettingen J, Sola Pou J, Levitsky LL, Misra M. Clinical presentation of children with premature adrenarche. Clin Pediatr (Phila). 2012;51(12):1140–9.

17. Martinez-Pajares JD, Diaz-Morales O, Ramos-Diaz JC, Gomez-Fernandez E. Peripheral precocious puberty due to inadvertent exposure to testosterone: case report and review of the literature. J Pediatr Endocrinol Metab. 2012;25:1007–12.

18. Healthy life chemistry by purity first B-50: FDA health risk warning—undeclared ingredients. 8-1-2013. (Internet Communication).

19. Diamanti-Kandarakis E, Bourguignon JP, Giudice LC, Hauser R, Prins GS, Soto AM, et al. Endocrine-disrupting chemicals: an Endocrine Society scientific statement. Endocr Rev. 2009;30(4):293–342.

20. State of the science: endocrine disrupting chemicals 2012. World Health Organization. 2012 (Internet Communication).

21. Wendt S, Shelso J, Wright K, Furman W. Neoplastic causes of abnormal puberty. Pediatr Blood Cancer. 2014;61(4):664–71.

22. Salpea P, Stratakis CA. Carney complex and McCune Albright syndrome: an overview of clinical manifestations and human molecular genetics. Mol Cell Endocrinol. 2014;386:85–91.

23. Bondy CA. Turner syndrome 2008. Horm Res. 2009;71 Suppl 1:52–6.

24. Kaufman FR, Kogut MD, Donnell GN, Goebelsmann U, March C, Koch R. Hypergonadotropic hypogonadism in female patients with galactosemia. N Engl J Med. 1981;304(17):994–8.

25. Cox L, Liu JH. Primary ovarian insufficiency: an update. Int J Womens Health. 2014;6:235–43.

26. Marsh CA, Auchus RJ. Fertility in patients with genetic deficiencies of cytochrome P450c17 (CYP17A1): combined 17-hydroxylase/17,20-lyase deficiency and isolated 17,20-lyase deficiency. Fertil Steril. 2014;101(2):317–22.

27. Velasco A, Vongpatanasin W. The evaluation and treatment of endocrine forms of hypertension. Curr Cardiol Rep. 2014;16(9):528.

28. Vongpatanasin W. Resistant hypertension: a review of diagnosis and management. JAMA. 2014;311(21):2216–24.
29. DiVasta AD, Gordon CM. Hormone replacement therapy and the adolescent. Curr Opin Obstet Gynecol. 2010;22(5):363–8.
30. Hardy TS, Norman RJ. Diagnosis of adolescent polycystic ovary syndrome. Steroids. 2013;78(8):751–4.
31. Azziz R. Controversy in clinical endocrinology: diagnosis of polycystic ovarian syndrome: the Rotterdam criteria are premature. J Clin Endocrinol Metab. 2006;91(3):781–5.
32. Azziz R, Carmina E, Dewailly D, Diamanti-Kandarakis E, Escobar-Morreale HF, Futterweit W, et al. The Androgen Excess and PCOS Society criteria for the polycystic ovarian syndrome: the complete task force report. Fertil Steril. 2009;91(2):456–8.
33. Bird ST, Hartzema AG, Etminan M, Brophy JM, Delaney JA. Polycystic ovary syndrome and combined oral contraceptive use: a comparison of clinical practice in the United States to treatment guidelines. Gynecol Endocrinol. 2013;29(4):365–9.
34. Bhattacharya SM, Jha A. Comparative study of the therapeutic effects of oral contraceptive pills containing desogestrel, cyproterone acetate, and drospirenone in patients with polycystic ovary syndrome. Fertil Steril. 2012;98(4):1053–9.
35. Manzoli L, De VC, Marzuillo C, Boccia A, Villari P. Oral contraceptives and venous thromboembolism: a systematic review and meta-analysis. Drug Saf. 2012;35(3):191–205.
36. Ehrmann DA, Liljenquist DR, Kasza K, Azziz R, Legro RS, Ghazzi MN. Prevalence and predictors of the metabolic syndrome in women with polycystic ovary syndrome. J Clin Endocrinol Metab. 2006;91(1):48–53.
37. TODAY Study Group. Safety and tolerability of the treatment of youth-onset type 2 diabetes: the TODAY experience. Diabetes Care. 2013;36(6):1765–71.

Chapter 7
Impact of Obesity on Female Puberty

Khalida Itriyeva and Ronald Feinstein

Abbreviations

BMI	Body mass index
DHEAS	Dehydroepiandrosterone sulfate
FSH	Follicle stimulating hormone
GnRH	Gonadotropin-releasing hormone
HOMA-IR	Homeostasis model assessment of IR
IR	Insulin resistance
LH	Luteinizing hormone
MCH	Melanin-concentrating hormone
NHANES	National Health and Nutrition Examination Survey
NPY	Neuropeptide Y

K. Itriyeva M.D. • R. Feinstein M.D., F.A.A.P.
Department of Adolescent Medicine, Cohen Children's
Medical Center of New York, 410 Lakeville Road Suite 108,
New Hyde Park, NY 11042, USA

© Springer International Publishing Switzerland 2016
H.L. Appelbaum (ed.), *Abnormal Female Puberty*,
DOI 10.1007/978-3-319-27225-2_7

PCOS	Polycystic ovary syndrome
SHBG	Sex hormone-binding globulin
YRBS	Youth Risk Behavior Surveillance

Introduction

Obesity in childhood and adolescence impacts normal female puberty, manifesting as earlier onset of puberty and irregularities of the menstrual cycle. Young obese girls presenting with thelarche before the expected age of 8 years should have a detailed history obtained with a focus on dietary assessment, as well as a physical exam performed including height, weight, and calculated body mass index. Additional history including evaluation for any neurologic or abdominal symptoms as well as family history regarding onset of puberty should be obtained. Labwork for the obese young child should include a routine complete blood count, comprehensive metabolic panel, hemoglobin A1c, and a lipid profile. Obese adolescents presenting with menstrual irregularities including anovulation or oligomenorrhea should have a detailed menstrual, sexual, and dietary history obtained, as well as a physical exam focused evaluation of body habitus, hirsutism, acne, acanthosis nigricans, alopecia, and an external genital exam. Laboratory evaluation should include a urine pregnancy test, luteinizing hormone, follicle stimulating hormone, estradiol, prolactin, thyroid studies, free and total testosterone, 17-hydroxyprogesterone, dehydroepiandrosterone sulfate, sex hormone-binding globulin, and hemoglobin A1c. Treatment of obesity should include nutrition counseling and encouragement of physical activity, with regular follow-up visits. Treatment of PCOS and associated menstrual irregularities is discussed in a separate chapter.

Case Presentation

A 10½-year-old African-American female presents to her pediatrician accompanied by her mother, who is concerned that her daughter has started menstruating. Menarche occurred 3 weeks ago and the patient's mother is worried that she is too young to be having her period, as the child is currently in fifth grade and none of her friends have begun menstruating yet. Maternal menarche occurred at age 13 and the patient's father reportedly developed at a similar age as his peers. Upon review of the patient's medical record, it is noted that thelarche occurred at age 8. Review of the stature-for-age growth chart reveals consistent growth at the 50th percentile until the past year, during which the child had a growth spurt. Upon review of the weight-for-age curve, it is noted that the patient was initially following the 50th percentile curve, but began to have accelerated weight gain starting at 4 years of age, and for the last 3 years has been above the 97th percentile.

Obtaining the social history reveals that the patient's family eats fast food or takeout most days of the week, as both parents work two jobs and do not have enough time to prepare meals at home. A 24 h food recall reveals a typical breakfast of an egg, cheese, and sausage sandwich, school lunch consisting of French fries and chicken nuggets with juice, an after-school snack of chips or cookies with whole milk, and fast food takeout for dinner. The patient does not engage in physical activity outside of school, but participates in physical education for 40 min 2–3 times per week. Review of systems is negative for headaches, seizures, visual changes, or abdominal pain. The patient does not take any medications or herbal supplements. Other than her obesity, she is healthy with no chronic medical problems or surgical history. Family history is notable for obesity and type 2 diabetes in the patient's father, paternal grandparents, and paternal aunt.

On physical examination, the patient's weight is 142 lb and height is 60 in., with a calculated body mass index (BMI) of 27.7. Acanthosis nigricans is noted on the neck. Heart, lung, abdomen, and neurologic exams, including fundoscopy, are normal. Breasts and pubic hair are both Sexual Maturity Rating (SMR) IV. There is no hirsutism. External genital exam reveals normal female genitalia without clitoromegaly. Laboratory tests including a complete blood count, comprehensive metabolic panel, and lipid profile are normal; however, hemoglobin A1c is noted to be in the prediabetic range. When plotted on the BMI-for-age CDC growth chart, the patient's BMI exceeds the 95th percentile based on her age and sex, thus classifying her as obese. A diet and exercise plan is discussed with the patient and her mother, and a follow-up appointment with the pediatrician and the office nutritionist is scheduled for the following month. The patient's mother is reassured that the cause of the patient's early pubertal development is likely her obesity.

Discussion

Childhood Obesity Definition and Epidemiology

Obesity in childhood is defined as a BMI at or above the 95th percentile based on sex-specific Centers for Disease Control (CDC) BMI-for-age growth charts [1, 2]. According to the Centers for Disease Control and Prevention and the National Health and Nutrition Examination Survey (NHANES) data from 2011 to 2012, the prevalence of childhood obesity remains high at 16.9 % for children ages 2–19 years with no significant overall change since 2003–2004 [1, 2]. Although the amount of obese 2- to 5-year-olds did decrease significantly between 2003 and 2004 and 2011–2012, from 13.9 to 8.4 %, the amount of obese adolescents remained relatively stable from 17.4 % in 2003–2004 to 20.5 % in 2011–2012, a change that was not statistically significant [2].

The prevalence of obesity is not equal among all youth, and disproportionally affects older children and adolescents, as well as minority racial groups. In the 2011–2012 NHANES survey, obesity rates were found to be higher in the older age groups, with only 8.4 % of 2- to 5-year-olds being classified as obese versus 17.7 % of 6- to 11-year-olds, and 20.5 % of 12- to 19-year-olds [2]. Obesity rates were also higher in minority youth, with 22.4 % of Hispanic children and 20.2 % of non-Hispanic black children meeting criteria for obesity, versus 14.1 % of non-Hispanic white children [2].

With childhood obesity rates having doubled in children and quadrupled in adolescents in the last 30 years [3], attention has focused on its prevention and treatment, as the short- and long-term health effects of childhood obesity are well documented and numerous. Short-term, obese children are more likely to suffer from hypertension, dyslipidemia, prediabetes, bone and joint problems, obstructive sleep apnea, and psychosocial consequences such as low self-esteem, bullying, and depression [4, 5]. Table 7.1 lists the multiple medical complications of childhood and adolescent obesity. The effects of these medical complications lead to a significantly lower health-related quality of life for obese children when compared to individuals of a healthy weight to a level that is comparable in children diagnosed with cancer [6]. Long-term, obese youth are more likely to become obese adults

Table 7.1 Medical complications of childhood and adolescent obesity

Neurologic

- Pseudotumor cerebri

Cardiovascular

- Hypertension
- Dyslipidemia

Endocrine

- Insulin resistance, impaired glucose tolerance, and type 2 diabetes
- Hyperandrogenism and PCOS
- Secondary amenorrhea
- Earlier onset of puberty

Gastrointestinal

- Nonalcoholic fatty liver disease
- Cholelithiasis

Pulmonary

- Obstructive sleep apnea
- Asthma

Orthopedic

- Slipped capital femoral epiphysis
- Blount disease

Psychosocial

- Depression
- Low self-esteem
- Stigmatization
- Eating disorders

[7]. Obesity in adulthood has further documented deleterious health effects including cardiovascular disease, type II diabetes, stroke, multiple types of cancer, and osteoarthritis [3, 8].

Factors Affecting Childhood and Adolescent Obesity

As obesity rates in youth have dramatically risen over the last 30 years, studies have begun to examine the various causes of obesity among children and adolescents. It appears that obesity is most likely a multifactorial disease with a complex interplay of genetics, diet, physical activity, and the environment playing a role in its development [4, 5, 8]. Among these factors, poor nutrition, a lack of physical activity, and the modern environment have had the greatest impact on the obesity epidemic. Table 7.2, adapted from Jasik and Lustig, summarizes the various risk factors for weight gain in adolescents.

Adolescence is a period of development when teenagers strive for autonomy and the ability to make their own decisions. However, when it comes to diet and nutrition, teenagers frequently make unhealthy choices. In the most recent Youth Risk Behavior Surveillance (YRBS) survey from 2013, only 21.9 % of high school students reported eating fruit or drinking 100 % fruit juice three or more times per day and only 15.7 % reported eating vegetables three or more times per day [9]. Furthermore, 19.4 % of students had not drunk milk in the 7 days prior to the survey, while 27 % of students reported drinking soda one or more times per day [9]. The food that teenagers do consume tends to be calorie rich and nutrient poor, and diets rich in high glycemic index foods and carbohydrates, saturated and trans fats, energy-dense foods, and sugar-sweetened beverages have contributed to the increased prevalence of obesity [4, 5, 8]. Increased consumption of these foods has resulted, in part, from the increased number of meals eaten outside the home in fast food chains and other restaurants [10], which also tend to serve larger portions.

Table 7.2 Psychosocial and behavioral risk factors for weight gain in early adolescence [8]

Risk factor	Examples
Sedentary lifestyle	Reduced physical education activities
	Less sports participation
	Less unstructured "play time"
	Increase in television viewing, computer use, and video game time
Overnutrition	Reduction in fruit and vegetable consumption
	More fast food consumption
	Increase in sweetened beverages, less milk consumption
	Higher overall calories consumed
Disordered eating/ obesogenic behavior	Skipping meals (e.g., breakfast)
	Fewer family meals
	Eating outside the home
	Dieting, binge eating, purging, taking laxatives/ diuretics
Mental health	Being teased or bullied
	Depression and anxiety
	Increased stress
	Psychotropic medication use
Built environment	School lunch and vending machines
	Neighborhood safety concerns
	Lack of available parks/recreation
	Fewer organized sports activities, school physical education
Developmental factors	Transitional cognitive development
	Increasing autonomy, less parental supervision
	Increases in peer influence
	Clustering of risk behaviors

Decreased physical activity and increased screen time with computers, video games, cell phones, and televisions have also contributed to the high rates of obesity among children and adolescents [4, 5, 8]. In the 2013 YRBS survey, only 27.1 % of students reported participating in at least 60 min of physical activity each day [9]. Just over 40 % of students reported playing video or computer games or using the computer for something other than school work for 3 or more hours per day and 32.5 % of students watched 3 or more hours of television per day [9]. Television viewing has not only been implicated as a sedentary behavior, but also in promoting weight gain due to children's passive consumption of energy-dense foods during their television viewing, and in showing commercials that advertise unhealthy foods and drinks [4, 11].

Children's home and school environments have also evolved over the last several decades, with greater access to television at home, less physical education classes in schools, and less after-school activities taking place outside [4]. Physical education (PE) in schools has been reduced for multiple reasons, and currently only 48 % of students report attending a PE class at least once a week and only 29.4 % report attending PE on every school day [9]. Children and adolescents are also consuming less meals at home and more meals at fast food restaurants. This shift over the last several decades has resulted in poorer nutrition for children, as family meals are associated with greater intake of fruits, vegetables, calcium, and vitamin-rich foods, and decreased intake of soft drinks [12].

In addition to the numerous environmental factors contributing to the high rates of childhood and adolescent obesity, genetics is also being studied and further appreciated as having a role in the development of obesity [13–15]. A systematic review of twin and adoption studies demonstrated that genetic factors have a strong effect on BMI [13]. It found that, while common environmental factors had an effect on BMI variation in children up to 13 years of age, after that age, this effect disappeared. In the adoption studies, strong correlations in weight were found between parents and their biological children. Additional research is currently being conducted on the genetics of obesity and, thus far, more than 200 obesity-associated genes have been discovered, in addition to specific single gene mutations and variants at particular loci that have also been shown to contribute to obesity [14, 15].

Obesity and Early Puberty

The timing of puberty and menarche in females is the result of a combination of genetic and environmental factors. In the last 200 years, there has been a trend towards earlier puberty, a result of better overall health and nutrition in women in industrialized countries [16]. However, in the past 30 years, girls have begun entering puberty and experiencing menarche at even younger ages [17]. As this phenomenon has occurred in parallel with the increased rates of childhood and adolescent obesity, it has been hypothesized that the earlier onset of puberty and menarche in girls is associated with overnutrition and adiposity [18].

Obesity appears to have a direct effect on the timing of puberty for girls, with earlier onset of both puberty and menarche seen in obese girls [17, 19]. The National Heart, Lung, and Blood Institute Growth and Health Study was a large-scale study that followed a group of girls annually for 10 years, from age 9 to 19, at three clinical centers across the country. They found that the mean age of menarche for Caucasian girls was 12.7 years, while the mean age for African-American girls was 12.0 years, with early maturing girls from both races having greater degrees of adiposity [20], and the racial differences being consistent with previous observations [21]. Researchers in 2001 further analyzed the data from the Pediatric Research in Office Settings (PROS) network [21], which showed that girls are entering puberty at earlier ages than previously described, and found that pubertal Caucasian girls ages 6–9 had significantly higher BMI z scores than prepubertal girls of the same age [18]. The same finding was seen for African-American girls, though to a lesser extent. Finally, the Bogalusa Heart Study investigated the secular trends in menarchal age in girls between 1973 and 1994 in a small community in Louisiana. During the 20-year study period, researchers found that the median menarchal age had decreased in African-American girls by approximately 9.5 months, from 12.9 to 12.1 years, and in Caucasian girls by 2 months, from 12.7 to 12.5 years [22]. Furthermore, more girls experienced early menarche, defined as <11.0 years old, a finding that was also more pronounced in African-American girls. Prevalence of early menarche increased from 5 to 17 % for

African-American girls and from 7 to 10 % for Caucasian girls during the 20-year period and was correlated with higher weights and BMIs [22]. A further study that investigated two cohorts in the Bogalusa Heart Study, one from 1978 to 1979 and another from 1992 to 1994, found that girls in the second cohort were heavier and had greater subscapular skinfold thickness than girls from the first cohort, and this was associated with the earlier onset of menarche seen in girls of the second cohort [23].

Chicken or the Egg?

The correlation between obesity and early puberty has forced researchers to ponder the question of which came first: does a high body fat mass predispose to early puberty, or does early puberty result in an increase in body fat? According to current research, it appears that the former is more accurate. Insulin resistance increases transiently during normal female puberty and is associated with a compensatory increase in insulin secretion, which likely contributes to the increase in body fat that occurs in females as they progress through puberty [24, 25]. Thus, girls entering puberty earlier may attain more body fat than their non-developed peers. However, studies have demonstrated that obese children going through puberty attain a higher degree of insulin resistance (IR) as expressed by the homeostasis model assessment of IR (HOMA-IR) than children of a normal weight [26, 27]. Thus, although a transient state of insulin resistance is normal during puberty, the phenomenon appears to be more pronounced in obese individuals and may contribute to further adiposity as well as increased risk of type 2 diabetes.

Studies have found that the weight status of girls in the years prior to onset of puberty affects the timing of puberty [28, 29]. A longitudinal study that followed 183 girls from age 5 to age 9 years found that girls with a higher percent body fat at age 5 years were more likely to have earlier onset of puberty by age 9 [28]. They also found that girls with a higher percent body fat, higher BMI percentile, and larger waist circumference at age 7 were more likely to be earlier developers at age 9. Finally, at age 9, the earlier developers had higher percent body fat, BMI percentiles, and waist circumferences than their non-developed peers. All associations between weight status at ages 5, 7, and 9 and timing of puberty at age 9 were independent of the girls' heights at these ages, thus pointing to a stronger association between adiposity and earlier puberty. Another longitudinal study several years later followed a cohort of 354 girls from the National Institute of Child Health and Human Development Study of Early Child Care and Youth Development [29]. The researchers measured the girls' height and weight at age 36, 54 months, and grades 1, 4, 5, and 6 and calculated BMI and BMI z scores at each age. Early puberty was defined in 4 ways: (1) breast development $\geq$Tanner 2 by physical examination at the grade 4 visit, (2) breast development $\geq$Tanner 3 by physical examination at the grade 5 visit, (3) maternal report of breast development $\geq$Tanner 3 at the grade 5 visit, and (4) maternal report of menarche having already occurred at the grade 6 visit. The investigators found that starting at age 36 months, a higher BMI z score at all the measured ages was strongly associated with an earlier onset of puberty. The researchers additionally found that the rate of BMI change between 36 months and first grade and accelerated BMI were also associated with earlier onset of puberty.

Thus, although early puberty appears to be associated with attainment of a higher body fat mass in females, it appears that greater adiposity in childhood predisposes females to earlier onset of puberty.

Obesity and Early Puberty: Physiology

The physiology of earlier onset of puberty as it relates to childhood obesity is complex and involves neuroendocrine pathways that are being elucidated by current research. Although the specifics of these pathways are not yet completely understood, it appears that a variety of hormones and peptides related to a state of adiposity are involved in sending signals to the prepubescent brain to initiate the pulsatile secretion of hypothalamic and pituitary hormones that mark the onset of puberty. Among these adiposity-related hormones, leptin has thus far been the most studied.

Leptin

Leptin is a hormone secreted by adipocytes and is the product of the obesity (ob) gene. Its role in appetite regulation has long been appreciated, but its additional role in puberty and human reproduction has been elucidated in recent years [30]. Obese children have higher serum leptin levels than children with normal BMIs [31], and are thus more likely to exhibit its effects.

Murine studies from the 1990s were the first to demonstrate the effects of leptin on reproductive function. The discovery of the *ob/ob* mouse, a mouse that is homozygous for the ob gene mutation and is unable to produce leptin, helped scientists uncover the important functions of leptin in appetite regulation and reproduction, as the *ob/ob* mice tended to be obese and infertile. A 1997 study by Chehab et al. also demonstrated the importance of leptin in mice without the mutation, as normal prepubertal female mice who were injected with human recombinant leptin were found to both reproduce earlier than controls and showed earlier maturation of their reproductive tracts [32]. Another study by the same lead author also revealed that administration of recombinant human leptin can correct the sterility of the homozygous female *ob/ob* mouse, allowing it to ovulate and become pregnant [33].

Subsequent human studies further uncovered the role of leptin in puberty and reproduction. A study of a consanguineous family with some members demonstrating a homozygous mutation in the human leptin receptor gene found that those members were both morbidly obese and had no spontaneous pubertal development, further alluding to the importance of leptin in endocrine and reproductive function [34]. Additionally, a study of 343 girls evaluating the effect of serum levels of leptin on menarche found that higher levels of leptin correlated with higher BMI and earlier age at menarche [35]. Specifically, the researchers discovered that, on average, each increase of 1 ng/mL in serum leptin decreased the timing of menarche by 1 month, and a gain of 1 kg in body fat decreased the menarchal age by approximately 13 days.

The specific neuroendocrine pathways by which leptin affects the onset of puberty and reproductive function are still being studied, but there is data to suggest that leptin acts at both the hypothalamic and pituitary levels. In one study involving a 9-year-old prepubertal, obese girl with congenital leptin deficiency, the administration of daily recombinant leptin therapy for 12 months resulted in weight loss, as well as pulsatile nighttime gonadotropin-releasing hormone (GnRH) secretion and increases in luteinizing hormone (LH) and follicle-stimulating hormone (FSH) suggestive of early puberty [36]. Leptin does appear to indirectly stimulate GnRH, as demonstrated by a study where rats who were administered leptin during a 48-h fast maintained a high LH pulse frequency, whereas those who were not given leptin had suppression of the LH pulse frequency [37]. Leptin also appears to affect reproductive function at the pituitary level, as demonstrated in a study by Yu et al., where hemi-anterior pituitaries of adult male rats were incubated with leptin and showed a dose-related increase in LH and FSH [38]. The results of this and other studies suggest that leptin, a hormone secreted by fat cells, provides information about the nutritional status of a mammal to the mechanisms that control the pulsatile release of GnRH. This mechanism is advantageous from an evolutionary standpoint as reproduction, pregnancy, and lactation all require great energy expenditure. The ability of female mammals to downregulate or turn off their reproductive systems at times of low food availability and resultant low body fat (and thus low leptin levels) is adaptive to reduce the female's risk of mortality from pregnancy and to reduce the chance that offspring are born into a resource-scarce environment where their survival may be difficult [17].

In spite of leptin's effects on the hypothalamus and pituitary, it is unlikely to be the primary signal that initiates puberty, but rather acts in a permissive fashion to allow puberty to occur under conditions when resources such as food are adequate [39]. This is supported by the fact that, although the presence of leptin stimulates GnRH release by the hypothalamus [40], it does not appear to act directly on GnRH neurons [41]. In the 2009 study by Quennell et al., mice with GnRH neuron-specific leptin receptor deletion demonstrated normal fertility, whereas those with forebrain neuron leptin receptor deletion did not undergo puberty and were infertile [41]. This finding suggests that other intermediate factors in the neuroendocrine pathway must be present and interact with leptin to stimulate the pulsatile GnRH release during puberty.

Intermediate Factors

The relationship between adiposity and the development of early puberty appears to be more complex, and is not solely explained by the higher levels of leptin in obese children undergoing earlier puberty. As previously mentioned, a complex interplay of hormones and other intermediate factors appears to be involved in the process.

Other intermediate factors that have been suggested in the activation of GnRH neurons include: ghrelin, neuropeptide Y (NPY), orexin, melanin-concentrating hormone (MCH), adiponectin, and kisspeptin [30]. The specific roles of these factors in puberty are beyond the scope of this chapter; however, an up-to-date overview is provided by Chehab in his article on leptin [30].

In addition to leptin and various intermediate factors, the insulin resistance and resultant compensatory hyperinsulinemia seen in obese children likely contribute to their earlier onset of puberty as well. The link between the effects of insulin on various organs and onset of puberty is summarized in Fig. 7.1, adapted from Ahmed et al. [19]. As the authors state, insulin resistance in obese children is associated with compensatory hyperinsulinemia and increased androgen production by the ovaries and adrenals, as well as decreased levels of sex hormone-binding globulin (SHBG), which results in increased sex steroid bioavailability. Additionally, increased adiposity results in increased conversion of androgens to estrogens through the action of aromatase, further contributing to the early onset and progression of puberty.

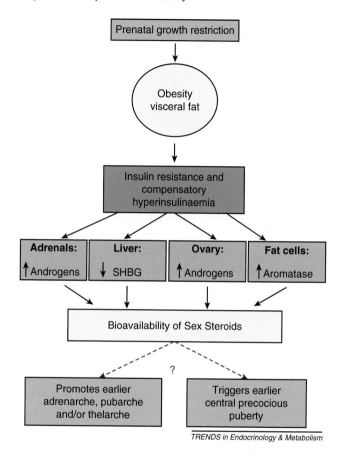

Fig. 7.1 Proposed endocrine pathways linking childhood obesity and insulin resistance to early pubertal onset and maturation [19]

Implications of Early Puberty in Females

Obesity has many short- and long-term implications for children and adolescents. However, early onset of puberty has significant psychosocial and medical implications for young females as well. From a psychosocial viewpoint, females who enter puberty at a young age are at higher risk for depression, anxiety, substance abuse, behavior problems, eating disorders, and promiscuity [42–45]. Medically, they are more likely to be heavier as adults [45]. Furthermore, studies have shown that girls with early menarche are at greater risk for type 2 diabetes and hypertension as adults, both risk factors for cardiovascular disease [46–48]. Breast cancer risk is also increased in girls with early menarche [49], and a recent meta-analysis found that overall mortality from all causes was higher in women who experienced early menarche [50].

Obesity and Menstrual Irregularities

In addition to experiencing earlier onset of puberty and menarche, obese girls are also at increased risk of hyperandrogenism and polycystic ovary syndrome (PCOS), and associated menstrual irregularities. PCOS and hyperandrogenism are discussed in detail in a separate chapter of this casebook, thus only a brief overview will be provided in this section.

Obesity is associated with hyperandrogenemia in young girls [51]. In their 2006 study, McCartney et al. evaluated 76 peripubertal girls ages 7–17, 35 of whom were normal weight and 41 of whom were obese. The researchers found that the obese girls, when compared to normal weight girls, had twice the level of total testosterone, 50 % lower SHBG, and triple the level of free testosterone [52]. Furthermore, mean fasting insulin levels were 50 % greater in obese girls than in normal weight girls. More importantly, upon analyzing only the girls in early puberty (Tanner stages 1–3), the researchers found that mean total testosterone levels were almost three times higher in obese girls than in normal weight girls. Additionally, SHBG was 50 % lower and free testosterone was five times higher in the obese young girls. The finding of this early onset of hyperandrogenemia is significant, as it can represent a precursor to PCOS.

Although obese girls are at increased risk for hyperandrogenemia, not all obese girls demonstrate the abnormal lab findings. To determine what factors may contribute to hyperandrogenemia in obese girls, Knudsen et al. studied 92 peripubertal obese girls at three separate sites in the United States [53]. The researchers measured the girls' LH, FSH, total and free testosterone, dehydroepiandrosterone (DHEAS), SHBG, fasting insulin, progesterone, and estradiol. They found that both morning levels of LH and fasting insulin were significant and independent predictors of free testosterone levels in their cohort of girls. Their findings suggest that both LH excess and hyperinsulinemia play a role in the development of hyperandrogenemia in obese girls.

The constellation of findings including insulin resistance with resultant hyperinsulinemia, hyperandrogenemia, and LH excess is that typically seen in girls and adult women with PCOS. PCOS has previously been defined in various ways, however, The Endocrine Society recommends using the Rotterdam criteria for diagnosis of PCOS, which requires that two of the following three criteria be met for the diagnosis to be established: (1) androgen excess as demonstrated by clinical or biochemical hyperandrogenism, (2) ovulatory dysfunction with oligo- or anovulation, and (3) polycystic ovaries on ultrasound, as defined by the presence of 12 or more follicles 2–9 mm in diameter and/or an increased ovarian volume >10 mL (without a cyst or dominant follicle) in either ovary [54]. Approximately 50 % of women with PCOS are obese [55], placing them at greater risk for insulin resistance and development of type 2 diabetes [54]. Diet, exercise, and medications such as metformin play an important role in the management of obese patients with PCOS to reduce their cardiovascular risk factors, and hormonal contraceptives are used as first-line therapy for treatment of the menstrual irregularities [54].

Obesity may also cause menstrual irregularities in adolescence as a result of disordered eating. Overweight girls are at higher risk for disordered eating including binge eating and extreme weight-control behaviors [56], which can affect the menstrual cycle. In addition to binge eating, they are also at risk for development of restrictive eating disorders and resultant amenorrhea [57]. Bulimia nervosa has also been associated with menstrual irregularities, particularly oligomenorrhea [58]. In studying patients with bulimia nervosa, Gendall et al. found additional factors that contributed to menstrual irregularities, including a higher frequency of vomiting, low levels of serum thyroxine, low dietary fat content, greater difference between maximum and minimum weight, and cigarette smoking [58].

Management

The treatment of childhood and adolescent obesity is often difficult, thus focus is placed on prevention, starting at birth. Expert committee recommendations published in Pediatrics in 2007 encourage primary care providers to provide counseling to children and their families regarding healthy eating habits and the importance of physical activity in obesity prevention [59]. The recommendations also stress the importance of measuring children's height, weight, and BMI at least annually, as well as performing a dietary assessment at each well-child visit and providing appropriate anticipatory guidance. Examples of nutritional recommendations include eating less meals outside the home and at fast food restaurants, reduction or elimination of sugar-sweetened beverage consumption, reduction of portion sizes, importance of consuming breakfast daily, and increasing intake of fruits and vegetables. The expert committee also recommends that providers assess physical activity and sedentary behaviors at each well-child visit, with counseling focused on encouraging at least 60 min of physical activity each day and no more than 2 h spent on sedentary behaviors. The provider should also assess the child's risk for comorbidities of obesity and inquire about family history of obesity, type 2 diabetes, cardiovascular disease, and early death from heart attack or stroke. In addition to performing a routine physical exam, the provider should also consider the following laboratory testing in a child with obesity: fasting lipid profile, AST, ALT, and fasting glucose levels. In terms of treatment, the expert committee recommends a staged approach, with four stages of increasing intensity focused on improving diet quality and increasing physical activity. The details of the four stages are outlined in the expert committee's summary report. The goals of therapy include development of permanent healthy lifestyle habits and reduction of BMI to <85th percentile, although some children may be healthy in the overweight category.

Outcome

The patient was followed by her pediatrician and a nutritionist every 2 weeks for the next 3 months. Dietary interventions included preparing more meals at home and consuming less fast food, consuming only skim and low-fat dairy products, eliminating sugar-sweetened beverages, decreasing consumption of energy-dense and fried food, and increasing intake of fruits and vegetables. In terms of physical activity, the patient joined a dance class 3 days per week in addition to her physical education class at school. Repeat hemoglobin A1c 3 months later was within normal limits, and the patient successfully lost 8 lb.

Conclusion

The obesity epidemic affecting children and adolescents in industrialized countries has numerous medical and psychosocial implications for youth, and affects their health as adults. For young girls, obesity is associated with earlier onset of puberty as well as menstrual irregularities. Research has focused on the mechanisms by which adiposity may cause early puberty, but the specific neuroendocrine pathways are still being elucidated through ongoing studies. The management of obesity and its comorbidities remains a challenge for physicians, with the mainstay of treatment focused on nutritional support and increased physical activity.

Clinical Pearls/Pitfalls

1. Higher prevalence of obesity in childhood has resulted in a secular trend towards earlier puberty in girls.
2. The increased prevalence of childhood obesity is due to a combination of poor diet, decreased physical activity, increased sedentary behaviors, social and environmental factors, and genetics.

146   K. Itriyeva and R. Feinstein

3. Earlier onset of puberty in obese girls is related to higher serum levels of leptin, which appears to act at the hypothalamic and pituitary level through intermediate factors.
4. Obese girls are at risk for hyperandrogenemia, insulin resistance, and menstrual irregularities which may result in development of PCOS.
5. Obesity prevention should be a part of every well-child visit; however, if a child is diagnosed as obese, a structured approach with nutritional counseling and physical activity recommendations must be undertaken.

References

1. Childhood obesity facts [Internet] 2014 Sep 3 [updated 2014 Sep 3; cited 2014 Nov 5]. http://www.cdc.gov/obesity/data/childhood.html.
2. Ogden CL, Carroll MD, Kit BK, Flegal KM. Prevalence of childhood and adult obesity in the United States, 2011-2012. JAMA. 2014;311(8):806–14.
3. Childhood obesity facts [Internet] 2014 Aug 13 [updated 2014 Aug 13; cited 2015 Jan 5]. http://www.cdc.gov/healthyyouth/obesity/facts.htm.
4. Ebbeling CB, Pawlak DB, Ludwig DS. Childhood obesity: public-health crisis, common sense cure. Lancet. 2002;360:473–82.
5. Jasik CB, Lustig RH. Adolescent obesity and puberty: the "perfect storm". Ann N Y Acad Sci. 2008;1135:265–79.
6. Schwimmer JB, Burwinkle TM, Varni JW. Health-related quality of life of severely obese children and adolescents. JAMA. 2003;289(14):1813–9.
7. Serdula MK, Ivery D, Coates RJ, Freedman DS, Williamson DF, Byers T. Do obese children become obese adults? A review of the literature. Prev Med. 1993;22(2):167–77.
8. Biro FM, Wien M. Childhood obesity and adult morbidities. Am J Clin Nutr. 2010;91(5):1499S–505.
9. Kann L, Kinchen S, Shanklin SL, Flint KH, Kawkins J, Harris WA, Lowry R, Olsen EO, McManus T, Chyen D, Whittle L, Taylor E, Demissie Z, Brener N, Thornton J, Moore J, Zaza S. Centers for Disease Control and Prevention (CDC). Youth risk behavior surveillance—United States, 2013. Morb Mortal Wkly Rep Surveill Summ. 2014;63 Suppl 4:1–168.
10. Bowman SA, Gortmaker SL, Ebbeling CB, Pereira MA, Ludwig DS. Effects of fast-food consumption on energy intake and diet quality among children in a national household survey. Pediatrics. 2004;113(1 Pt 1):112–8.
11. Borzekowski DL, Robinson TN. The 30-second effect: an experiment revealing the impact of television commercials on food preferences of preschoolers. J Am Diet Assoc. 2001;101(1):42–6.

12. Neumark-Sztainer D, Hannan PJ, Story M, Croll J, Perry C. Family meal patterns: associations with sociodemographic characteristics and improved dietary intake among adolescents. J Am Diet Assoc. 2003;103(3):317–22.
13. Silventoinen K, Rokholm B, Kaprio J, Sorensen TIA. The genetic and environmental influences on childhood obesity: a systematic review of twin and adoption studies. Int J Obes (Lond). 2009;34:29–40.
14. Rankinen T, Zuberi A, Chagnon YC, Weisnagel SJ, Argyropoulos G, Walts B, Perusse L, Bouchard C. The human obesity gene map: the 2005 update. Obesity. 2006;14(4):529–644.
15. Ntalla I, Panoutsopoulou K, Vlachou P, Southam L, William Rayner N, Zeggini E, Dedoussis GV. Replication of established common genetic variants for adult BMI and childhood obesity in Greek adolescents: the TEENAGE study. Ann Hum Genet. 2013;77(3):268–74.
16. Ong KK, Ahmed ML, Dunger DB. Lessons from large population studies on timing and tempo of puberty (secular trends and relation to body size): the European trend. Mol Cell Endocrinol. 2006;254-255:8–12.
17. Kaplowitz PB. Link between body fat and the timing of puberty. Pediatrics. 2008;121 Suppl 3:S208–17.
18. Kaplowitz PB, Slora EJ, Wasserman RC, Pedlow SE, Herman-Giddens ME. Earlier onset of puberty in girls: relation to increased body mass index and race. Pediatrics. 2001;108(2):347–53.
19. Ahmed ML, Ong KK, Dunger DB. Childhood obesity and the timing of puberty. Trends Endocrinol Metab. 2009;20(5):237–42.
20. Biro FM, McMahon RP, Striegel-Moore R, Crawford PB, Obarzanek E, Morrison JA, Barton BA, Falkner F. Impact of timing of pubertal maturation on growth in black and white female adolescents: The National Heart, Lung, and Blood Institute Growth and Health Study. J Pediatr. 2001;138(5):636–43.
21. Herman-Giddens ME, Slora EJ, Wasserman RC, Bourdony CJ, Bhapkar MV, Koch GG, Hasemeier CM. Secondary sexual characteristics and menses in young girls seen in office practice: a study from the Pediatric Research in Office Settings network. Pediatrics. 1997;99(4):505–12.
22. Freedman DS, Kettel Khan L, Serdula MK, Dietz WH, Srinivasan SR, Berenson GS. Relation of age at menarche to race, time period, and anthropometric dimensions: the Bogalusa heart study. Pediatrics. 2002;4:110(4). Available at: www.pediatrics.org/cgi/content/full/110/4/e43.
23. Wattigney WA, Srinivasan SR, Chen W, Greenlund KJ, Berenson GS. Secular trend of earlier onset of menarche with increasing obesity in black and white girls: the Bogalusa Heart Study. Ethn Dis. 1999 Spring-Summer;9(2):181–9.
24. Moran A, Jacobs Jr DR, Steinberger J, Hong CP, Prineas R, Luepker R, Sinaiko AR. Insulin resistance during puberty: results from clamp studies in 357 children. Diabetes. 1999;48(10):2039–44.
25. Caprio S, Plewe G, Diamond MP, Simonson DC, Boulware SD, Sherwin RS, Tamborlane WV. Increased insulin secretion in puberty: a compensatory response to reductions in insulin sensitivity. J Pediatr. 1989;114(6):963–7.

26. Pilia S, Casini MR, Foschini ML, Minerba L, Musiu MC, Marras V, Civolani P, Loche S. The effect of puberty on insulin resistance in obese children. J Endocrinol Invest. 2009;32(5):401–5.

27. Pinhas-Hamiel O, Lerner-Geva L, Copperman NM, Jacobson MS. Lipid and insulin levels in obese children: changes with age and puberty. Obesity. 2007;15(11):2825–31.

28. Davison KK, Susman EJ, Birch LL. Percent body fat at age 5 predicts earlier pubertal development among girls at age 9. Pediatrics. 2003;111(4 Pt 1): 815–21.

29. Lee JM, Appugliese D, Kaciroti N, Corwyn RF, Bradley RH, Lumeng JC. Weight status in young girls and the onset of puberty. Pediatrics. 2007;119(3):e624–30.

30. Chehab FF. 20 years of leptin: leptin and reproduction: past milestones, present undertakings, and future endeavors. J Endocrinol. 2014;223(1):T37–48.

31. Hassink SG, Sheslow DV, de Lancey E, Opentanova I, Considine RV, Caro JF. Serum leptin in children with obesity: relationship to gender and development. Pediatrics. 1996;98(2 Pt 1):201–3.

32. Chehab FF, Mounzih K, Lu R, Lim ME. Early onset of reproductive function in normal female mice treated with leptin. Science. 1997;275(5296):88–90.

33. Chehab FF, Lim ME, Lu R. Correction of the sterility defect in homozygous obese female mice by treatment with the human recombinant leptin. Nat Genet. 1996;12(3):318–20.

34. Clement K, Vaisse C, Lahlou N, Cabrol S, Pelloux V, Cassuto D, Gourmelen M, Dina C, Chambaz J, Lacorte JM, Basdevant A, Bougneres P, Lebouc Y, Froguel P, Guy-Grand B. A mutation in the human leptin receptor gene causes obesity and pituitary dysfunction. Nature. 1998;392(6674):398–401.

35. Matkovic V, Ilich JZ, Skugor M, Badenhop NE, Goel P, Clairmont A, Klisovic D, Nahhas RW, Landoll JD. Leptin is inversely related to age at menarche in human females. J Clin Endocrinol Metab. 1997;82(10):3239–45.

36. Farooqi IS, Jebb SA, Langmack G, Lawrence E, Cheetham CH, Prentice AM, Hughes IA, McCamish MA, O'Rahilly S. Effects of recombinant leptin therapy in a child with congenital leptin deficiency. N Engl J Med. 1999;341(12):879–84.

37. Nagatani S, Guthikonda P, Thompson RC, Tsukamura H, Maeda KI, Foster DL. Evidence for GnRH regulation by leptin: leptin administration prevents reduced pulsatile LH secretion during fasting. Neuroendocrinology. 1998;67(6):370–6.

38. Yu WH, Kimura M, Walczewska A, Karanth S, McCann SM. Role of leptin in hypothalamic-pituitary function. Proc Natl Acad Sci U S A. 1997;94(3): 1023–8.

39. Cheung CC, Thornton JE, Kuijper JL, Weigle DS, Clifton DK, Steiner RA. Leptin is a metabolic gate for the onset of puberty in the female rat. Endocrinology. 1997;138(2):855–8.

40. Reynoso R, Ponzo OJ, Szwarcfarb B, Rondina D, Carbone S, Rimoldi G, Scacchi P, Moguilevsky JA. Effect of leptin on hypothalamic release of GnRH and neurotransmitter amino acids during sexual maturation in female rats. Exp Clin Endocrinol Diabetes. 2003;111(5):274–7.

41. Quennell JH, Mulligan AC, Tups A, Liu X, Phipps SJ, Kemp CJ, Herbison AE, Grattan DR, Anderson GM. Leptin indirectly regulates gonadotropin-releasing hormone neuronal function. Endocrinology. 2009;150(6):2805–12.
42. Lee Y, Styne D. Influences on the onset and tempo of puberty in human beings and implications for adolescent psychological development. Horm Behav. 2013;64(2):250–61.
43. Kaltiala-Heino R, Kosunen E, Rimpela M. Pubertal timing, sexual behaviour and self-reported depression in middle adolescence. J Adolesc. 2003;26(5):531–45.
44. Zehr JL, Culbert KM, Sisk CL, Klump KL. An association of early puberty with disordered eating and anxiety in a population of undergraduate women and men. Horm Behav. 2007;52(4):427–35.
45. Johansson T, Ritzen EM. Very long-term follow-up of girls with early and late menarche. Endocr Dev. 2005;8:126–36.
46. Mueller NT, Duncan BB, Barreto SM, Chor D, Bessel M, Aquino EM, Pereira MA, Schmidt MI. Earlier age at menarche is associated with higher diabetes risk and cardiometabolic disease risk factors in Brazilian adults: Brazilian Longitudinal Study of Adult Health (ELSA-Brasil). Cardiovasc Diabetol. 2014;13:22.
47. Dreyfus JG, Lutsey PL, Huxley R, Pankow JS, Selvin E, Fernandez-Rhodes L, Franceschini N, Demerath EW. Age at menarche and risk of type 2 diabetes among African-American and white women in the Atherosclerosis Risk in Communities (ARIC) study. Diabetologia. 2012;55(9):2371–80.
48. Lakshman R, Forouhi NG, Sharp SJ, Luben R, Bingham SA, Khaw KT, Wareham NJ, Ong KK. Early age at menarche associated with cardiovascular disease and mortality. J Clin Endocrinol Metab. 2009;94(12): 4953–60.
49. Velie EM, Nechuta S, Osuch JR. Lifetime reproductive and anthropometric risk factors for breast cancer in postmenopausal women. Breast Dis. 2005–2006;24:17–35.
50. Charalampopoulos D, McLoughlin A, Elks CE, Ong KK. Age at menarche and risks of all-cause and cardiovascular death: a systematic review and meta-analysis. Am J Epidemiol. 2014;180(1):29–40.
51. McCartney CR, Blank SK, Prendergast KA, Chhabra S, Eagleson CA, Helm KD, Yoo R, Chang RJ, Foster CM, Caprio S, Marshall JC. Obesity and sex steroid changes across puberty: evidence for marked hyperandrogenemia in pre- and early pubertal obese girls. J Clin Endocrinol Metab. 2007;92(2):430–6.
52. McCartney CR, Prendergast KA, Chhabra S, Eagleson CA, Yoo R, Chang RJ, Foster CM, Marshall JC. The association of obesity and hyperandrogenemia during the pubertal transition in girls: obesity as a potential factor in the genesis of postpubertal hyperandrogenism. J Clin Endocrinol Metab. 2006;91(5):1714–22.
53. Knudsen KL, Blank SK, Burt Solorzano C, Patrie JT, Chang RJ, Caprio S, Marshall JC, McCartney CR. Hyperandrogenemia in obese peripubertal girls: correlates and potential etiological determinants. Obesity (Silver Spring). 2010;18(11):2118–24.

54. Legro RS, Arslanian SA, Ehrmann DA, Hoeger KM, Murad MH, Pasquali R, Welt CK. Endocrine Society. Diagnosis and treatment of polycystic ovary syndrome: an Endocrine Society clinical practice guideline. J Clin Endocrinol Metab. 2013;98(12):4565–92.
55. Azziz R, Sanchez LA, Knochenhauer ES, Moran C, Lazenby J, Stephens KC, Taylor K, Boots LR. Androgen excess in women: experience with over 1000 consecutive patients. J Clin Endocrinol Metab. 2004;89(2): 453–62.
56. Neumark-Sztainer DR, Wall MM, Haines JI, Story MT, Sherwood NE, van den Berg PA. Shared risk and protective factors for overweight and disordered eating in adolescents. Am J Prev Med. 2007;33(5):359–69.
57. Lebow J, Sim LA, Kransdorf LN. Prevalence of a history of overweight and obesity in adolescents with restrictive eating disorders. J Adolesc Health. 2015;56(1):19–24.
58. Gendall KA, Bulik CM, Joyce PR, McIntosh VV, Carter FA. Menstrual cycle irregularity in bulimia nervosa: Associated factors and changes with treatment. J Psychosom Res. 2000;49(6):409–15.
59. Barlow SE, Committee E. Expert committee recommendations regarding the prevention, assessment, and treatment of child and adolescent overweight and obesity: summary report. Pediatrics. 2007;120 Suppl 4:S164–92.

Chapter 8
Anorexia Nervosa in the Young Female Adolescent

Martin Fisher and Alexis Santiago

Abbreviations

APA   American Psychiatric Association
FSH   Follicle-stimulating hormone
GH   Growth hormone
GnRH   Gonadotropin-releasing hormone
IGF-1   Insulin growth factor 1
LH   Luteinizing hormone

M. Fisher, M.D. (✉)
Division of Adolescent Medicine, Cohen Children's Medical Center,
Northwell Health System, 410 Lakeville Road, Suite 108,
New Hyde Park, NY 11042, USA

Hofstra Northwell School of Medicine,
Hempstead, NY, USA
e-mail: fisher@nshs.edu

A. Santiago, M.D.
Division of Adolescent Medicine, Cohen Children's Medical Center,
Northwell Health System, 410 Lakeville Road, Suite 108,
New Hyde Park, NY 11042, USA
e-mail: asantiag13@nshs.edu

© Springer International Publishing Switzerland 2016
H.L. Appelbaum (ed.), *Abnormal Female Puberty*,
DOI 10.1007/978-3-319-27225-2_8

Introduction

The eating disorders, anorexia nervosa and related conditions, represent one of the major causes of abnormal female puberty in contemporary society. Anorexia nervosa is reported to occur in 0.5 % of adolescent females, the third most common chronic disease in teenage girls, after asthma and obesity [1]. Original reports indicated that there was a bi-model distribution of anorexia nervosa in adolescents, with peaks in both early and late adolescence, but more recent evidence indicates it is relatively equally distributed throughout the adolescent years. Females represent 90 % of cases, with a recent increase in cases reported in males due to the greater attention males have paid to body image concerns in the past 15 years and an increased focus on "healthy eating" showed by both female and male adolescents [2]. When anorexia nervosa occurs in the pre- or peri-pubertal female adolescent, there are specific issues in diagnosis, medical complications, evaluation, and treatment that require special attention. These issues will be reviewed in this chapter.

Case Presentation

A 14-year-old female was seen for a follow-up of protein calorie malnutrition secondary to anorexia nervosa, restricting type. She initially presented to the office at age 11, with concerns of poor eating and a 15 lb weight loss in a 4-month period. She had no significant past medical history. Her maximum weight had been 78 lb about 5 months earlier. She reported that she initially wanted to "be healthy" and decreased her portion sizes and avoided junk food. She gradually became more restrictive, eventually eliminating gluten and becoming a vegetarian. In addition to restricting, she exercised by running 3 miles 5 times a week. At the time, she did not have a personal weight goal but wanted to appear "healthy."

At her initial visit, the patient's weight was 65 lb, in the 10th percentile, and her height was 57 in., in the 52nd percentile. Her body mass index (BMI) was 14.1, which placed her in the 2nd percentile for BMI (see attached growth curves, Figs. 8.1 and 8.2). Her

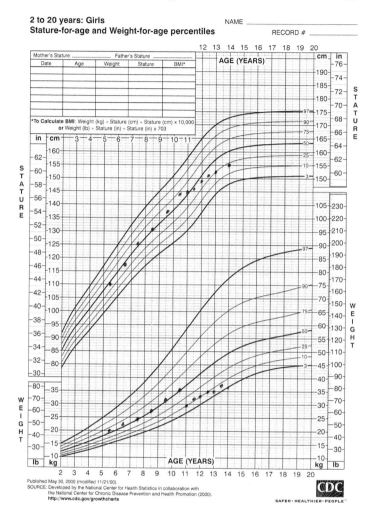

Fig. 8.1 2–20 Years: girls stature-for-age and weight-for-age percentiles

vital signs were within normal limits and she did not have bradycardia. Her physical examination was consistent with a pre-pubertal
female with a sexual maturity rating (SMR) of one for both breasts
and pubic hair. The remainder of the physical examination was
unremarkable. Laboratory testing was obtained (complete blood

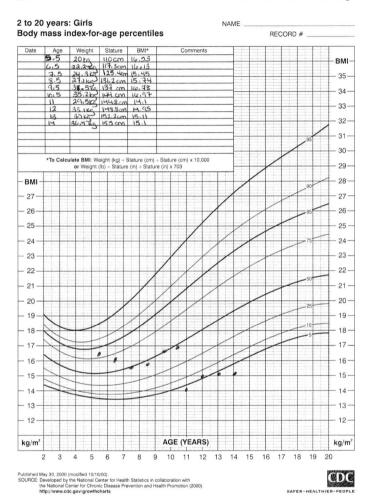

2 to 20 years: Girls
Body mass index-for-age percentiles

NAME _____

RECORD # _____

Date	Age	Weight	Stature	BMI*	Comments
	5.5	20 kg	110 cm	16.53	
	6.5	22.3 kg	117.3 cm	16.13	
	7.5	24.3 kg	125.4 cm	15.45	
	8.5	27.1 kg	131.2 cm	15.74	
	9.5	31.5 kg	137 cm	16.78	
	10.5	35.2 kg	144 cm	16.97	
	11	29.5 kg	144.8 cm	14.1	
	12	35.1 kg	148.8 cm	14.95	
	13	35 kg	152.2 cm	15.11	
	14	36.4 kg	155 cm	15.1	

*To Calculate BMI: Weight (kg) ÷ Stature (cm) ÷ Stature (cm) x 10,000
or Weight (lb) ÷ Stature (in) ÷ Stature (in) x 703

Published May 30, 2000 (modified 10/16/00).
SOURCE: Developed by the National Center for Health Statistics in collaboration with
the National Center for Chronic Disease Prevention and Health Promotion (2000).
http://www.cdc.gov/growthcharts

Fig. 8.2 2 to 20 Years: girls body mass index-for-age percentiles

count, complete metabolic panel, thyroid function tests, celiac panel, and erythrocyte sedimentation rate) and all tests were within normal limits.

She continued to follow up at the office inconsistently for the next 3 years. She continued to be fearful of and resistant to weight gain. Throughout her treatment, it was recommended that she receive a higher level of care, such as an admission to a day program or a residential facility; however, her parents were not agreeable because they did not want her to be away from home. She saw several therapists sporadically throughout the 3 years and her family considered family-based therapy at one point but felt they would not be able to implement the parental controls required by that approach. The patient did have some times during the 3 years where her eating disorder thoughts were a little better and she was able to reach a maximum weight of 82 lb when she was 13.5 years of age. She denies exercising but her parents suspect she does exercise when she is not being supervised. Based on her dietary recall, it is estimated that she is eating approximately 1400 cal per day.

At age 14 years, she remains premenarchal. Maternal menarche was at age 16 years and while the maternal history is not explicitly notable for an eating disorder, the patient's mother commented that women in the family tend to be thin and "have later periods."

On examination, the patient weighs 80 lb, in the 3rd percentile, and her height is 61 in., in the 20th percentile. Her BMI is 15.1, placing her in the 1st percentile for BMI (Figs. 8.1 and 8.2). Her vital signs are within normal limits. Her physical examination is notable for absence of breast budding or pubic hair but is otherwise unremarkable. Laboratory tests are again obtained and are notable for a low T3 (0.4 ng/mL) but a normal T4 (1.12 ng/ml and TSH (4 µIU/mL)). Her estradiol is <10 pg/mL, with a lutenizing hormone (LH) of <0.1 IU/L, follicle-stimulating hormone (FSH) of 1.18 IU/L, and a normal prolactin of 5.2 ng/ml.

Discussion

The patient was diagnosed as having anorexia nervosa on her initial presentation as an 11-year-old and she still has this diagnosis as a 14-year-old. The effect of on-going malnutrition on her growth and development, and her lack of menarche by age 14, exemplifies a major medical complication of the disorder specific to the young adolescent female. Her resistance to treatment, along with her family's inability and/or unwillingness to take the steps necessary to bring about her recovery, demonstrates important issues encountered in the treatment of patients with eating disorders in this age group.

Diagnosis

For the past four decades, the diagnosis of eating disorders, as well as other psychiatric conditions, has followed the guidelines established by the *Diagnostic and Statistical Manual* (DSM) published by the American Psychiatric Association (APA). The fourth edition of the DSM (DSM-IV) was published in 1990 [3], and the criteria for all psychiatric diagnoses, including those of the eating disorders, were listed in the DSM-IV (and a revision, the DSM-IV-TR, published in 1994) from then until the publication of the 5th edition of the DSM (DSM-5) in May of 2013 [4]. The introduction of the DSM-5 brought about major changes in the criteria of almost all psychiatric diagnoses, with the changes in the diagnosis of anorexia nervosa and other eating disorders being especially helpful in establishing criteria that more accurately reflect the most appropriate diagnoses in all age groups, especially children and peri-pubertal adolescents. The DSM-IV contained three specific eating disorder diagnoses: anorexia nervosa, bulimia nervosa, and "eating disorder not otherwise specified" (EDNOS), the latter being a catch-all category to describe those who had an obvious eating disorder but who did not fit the specific criteria established for the diagnoses of anorexia nervosa (AN) or bulimia nervosa (BN). In order to have a DSM-IV diagnosis of AN, four criteria needed to be met. These were that the patient had:

1. Refusal to maintain body weight at or above a minimally normal weight for age and height (e.g., weight loss leading to maintenance of body weight less than 85 % of that expected or failure to make expected weight gain during a period of growth, leading to body weight less than 85 % of that expected).
2. Intense fear of gaining weight or becoming fat, even though underweight.

3. Distortion in the way in which one's body weight or shape is experienced,
4. In post menarcheal females, amenorrhea (i.e., the absence of at least three consecutive menstrual cycles).

In order to have a DSM-IV diagnosis of BN, five criteria were required. These were:

1. Recurrent episodes of binge eating.
2. Recurrent inappropriate compensatory behaviors in order to prevent weight gain, such as self-induced vomiting, misuse of laxatives, diuretics, enemas, or other medications; fasting; or excessive exercise.
3. The binge eating and inappropriate compensatory behaviors both occur on average twice a week.
4. Self-evaluation is unduly influenced by body-shape and weight.
5. The disturbance does not occur exclusively during episodes of anorexia nervosa.

Patients who did not meet these specific criteria for AN or BN were given a DSM-IV diagnosis of EDNOS.

The criteria specify that in order for there to be a diagnosis of AN, there must be fear of weight gain and/or distortion of body image. This can be expressed in different ways, and is often initially denied by patients, especially older children and younger adolescents, but fear of weight gain and/or body image distortion must be present for there to be a diagnosis of AN. Other causes for the poor eating and/or weight loss can lead to alternate eating disorder diagnoses which have been introduced in the DSM-5, or to other medical or psychiatric diagnoses that must be considered in the differential diagnosis. The patient in the vignette initially expressed her decreased intake and increased exercise as a desire to "be healthy," which has become the most frequent terminology used by patients with AN in recent years (as compared to the patients in the 1980s who mostly said they had "eliminated carbohydrates" from their diets and the patients in the 1990s who said they had "eliminated fats"), but her unwillingness to make changes that would lead to weight gain ultimately confirmed the diagnosis of anorexia nervosa.

The DSM-IV diagnosis of AN stipulated that the patient had to be at least 15 % below her expected body weight in order to meet the required criteria. While the term "expected body weight" is no longer utilized (implying that there is a single expected weight for each person based on their gender, age, and height) and is increasingly being replaced by the term "average body weight" (implying that there is a single number representing an average for a particular gender, age and height), the concept was found to have both positive and negative utility. On the positive side, the ability to do a calculation that compares an individual's weight to an average for her age and height does provide one useful indicator of severity. The most formal way to perform this calculation at present is to determine the 50th percentile for BMI for the individuals' age and gender (as seen in the Centers for Disease Control and Prevention (CDC) BMI curve for females presented in Fig. 8.2), to determine the weight that BMI requires, and to then calculate a percentage comparing these two numbers. A simpler way to calculate this clinically is to use the mnemonic "the average weight for a female who is 5 ft tall is 100 lb and the average increase is 5 lb for every inch above that." This calculation comes out to be very close to the calculation performed more formally, with younger adolescents being a few pounds below the calculated number and older adolescents being a few pounds above. Thus, in the DSM-IV criteria it was required that the individual be at least 15 % below the established average; so, for instance, a 16-year-old female at 64″ would need to be 102 lb or below (since 18 lb is 15 % below the 120 lb average for her height) to meet the official criteria. The negative of using the strict number of 15 % meant that individuals who did not meet this criteria, such as those who started out very overweight and had lost a lot of weight but were still overweight, and who had significant psychological and physical indications of an eating disorder, could not receive a diagnosis of anorexia nervosa. In our own eating disorder treatment program for adolescents, we had almost as many patients over the years in this latter category as we did patients who became 15 % below average weight for height [5].

One other problem with the 15 % below average criteria, which applies particularly to pre- and peri-pubertal patients, was acknowledged and handled well in the DSM-IV criteria. Specifically, the criteria acknowledged that since both weight and height could be affected by the malnutrition caused by AN, a younger patient could meet the criteria by being 15 % below what her weight should have been. For younger patients, growth curves for both weight and height should be used to determine what the patient's weight and height potentially would have been if they had not restricted their caloric intake.

The fourth criteria for the diagnosis of AN in the DSM-IV was the absence of menstruation for at least 3 months. In the context of the pre-pubertal patient, several points regarding this criteria are important to note. First, there are clearly some patients who present for the evaluation of anorexia nervosa before they have lost three periods, and thus these patients would be technically eliminated from having a diagnosis of AN even if they met all other criteria. Second, for those patients not expected to have periods, such as those who are premenarchal (or boys) this criteria did not eliminate those patients from the diagnosis. Third, although many studies indicated that most girls and women would lose their periods when they are approximately 13–15 % below average body weight, this is far from universal and initial weight (not just a comparison to the average for age and height) must also be taken into account. Lastly, many early studies found that some patients become amenorrheic even before they have any weight loss, with no specific explanation ever determined for this finding [6].

In terms of bulimia nervosa, it should be noted that this diagnosis is more common in college age and young adult women (estimated to be 1–3 % in these populations) than it is in adolescents [7, 8]. It is rare in young adolescents, but not nonexistent. The guidelines for BN in the DSM-IV included the criteria that referred to binge eating, which is much more common in young adults with purging behaviors than in adolescents who purge. Another criteria referred to compensatory behaviors that would cause weight loss (such as vomiting, laxatives use, excessive exercise, or periods of relative starvation), without which the patients would have binge-eating disorder and subsequent obesity. And one criteria indicated that, as in AN, the patient with BN (who could be underweight, normal weight, or overweight) had to be participating in her eating disorder behaviors because of concerns with weight and/or body image [3].

According to the DSM-IV criteria, those patients who did not meet the strict criteria for AN or BN were given the diagnosis of

EDNOS. We determined in a study of 309 children and adolescents presenting to our program from September 2011 through December 2012 that 64 % of our patients had a diagnosis of EDNOS [5]. This included mostly patients who did not meet the criteria of falling to 15 % below average weight (most of whom were overweight initially and were still overweight despite significant weight loss at presentation), some patients who had not had amenorrhea for 3 months, some patients who did not meet criteria for BN because they were purging but did not binge, and some patients who ate poorly and lost weight or did not grow appropriately because of reasons other than fear of weight gain or body image issues.

The predominance of EDNOS diagnoses was the major focus of the Eating Disorder Work Group assigned by the APA to establish the new eating disorder criteria for the DSM-5 [4]. In response, they made several specific changes, with excellent results: (1) For the diagnosis of AN, the DSM-5 criteria no longer require a specific weight percent that patients must be below (although still indicating that for a diagnosis of AN the patient does have to be underweight); the criteria of amenorrhea were eliminated totally (with the logic being that amenorrhea is a physiologic response to malnutrition, not a core psychiatric feature of the illness, and the DSM is a psychiatric compendium); and a new subcategory of Atypical Anorexia Nervosa was added (to include those patients who started out obese and were still overweight, but had developed an eating disorder in the course of their dieting and weight loss). (2) For the diagnosis of bulimia nervosa, the DSM-5 decreased the required frequency of binging and purging from at least twice a week to at least once a week (which has not had a significant effect on total diagnoses); made binge-eating disorder an official diagnosis (which has had almost no effect on the adolescent age group, and especially the young adolescent age group, since almost all binge-eating disorder diagnoses occur in adults); and most importantly for the adolescent age group, added an official diagnosis of purging disorder, which now incorporates the many adolescents, including some young adolescents, who purge but do not binge. (3) The DSM-5 also now includes a new diagnosis entitled Avoidant-Restrictive Food Intake Disorder (ARFID). This diagnosis, based on a previous DSM-IV diagnosis that applied only to children 6 years of age or below, includes all of those children and adolescents who do not eat well and have poor growth or weight loss but who do not have a fear of weight gain or body image concerns. This is a particularly important diagnosis for pre- and peri-pubertal children and adolescents. In one study of 98 patients with the newly described diagnosis of ARFID seen in seven adolescent eating disorder programs in the United States and Canada, the mean age of the patients was 12.9 years, with patients having poor eating either because of (a) a choking or vomiting episode that led to fear of eating solid foods, (b) a very restricted diet from a very young age, (c) abdominal symptoms (usually due to irritable bowel syndrome) leading to decreased eating (which would then lead to more abdominal symptoms in an on-going cycle), or (d) generalized anxiety that led to decreased appetite [9].

In total, the switch from the DSM-IV to the DSM-5 criteria in 2013 has had a major effect on the diagnosis of eating disorders, especially anorexia nervosa, in the adolescent age group, and especially in young adolescents. Among the 309 patients in our program described earlier as having 64 % of patients placed in the DSM-IV category of EDNOS, these same patients all have specific diagnoses (with the exception of 4 patients who could not be categorized) according to the new DSM-5 criteria [5]. Specifically, while there were 80 patients with AN, 29 with BN, and 198 with EDNOS using the DSM-IV criteria, these same patients are now categorized by the DSM-5 criteria as 100 patients with AN, 80 patients with atypical AN, 29 with BN, 19 with purging disorder, and 60 (almost 20 % of the total) with ARFID [5]. In the context of this chapter on the peri-pubertal female, it is the latter finding that may be most important, as it is critical to distinguish between those older children and younger adolescents who present with poor eating and weight loss or poor growth who have anorexia nervosa (marked by fear of weight gain and body image issues) and those who have ARFID (and thus have other reasons for their poor nutritional intake). The patient in the vignette does, in fact, have a diagnosis of anorexia nervosa and not ARFID, as was clear on her presentation and became ever more clear as her fear of weight gain became even more obvious as time went on.

Medical Complications

As would be expected, the medical complications found in patients
with eating disorders occur in a wide range of organ systems. In the
case of anorexia nervosa, the medical findings are caused by malnutrition. In the case of bulimia nervosa they are caused by the
compensatory behaviors (such as vomiting or laxative use) utilized
by the patient as a method of weight control in addition to the
results of malnutrition. Most of the medical complications of eating
disorders occur similarly in all age groups, including peri-pubertal
adolescents, but one set of problems, primary amenorrhea and
delays in growth and development, are specific to this age group.
The medical findings (including weight loss or vomiting) found in
patients with eating disorders can certainly also be found in many
other medical (and psychiatric) conditions. Thus, it is important to
consider these other medical disorders (including inflammatory
bowel disease or celiac disease, hypo- or hyper-thyroidism, diabetes mellitus or insipidus, and brain tumors or other occult malignancies) and/or psychiatric disorders (including depression,
anxiety, obsessive-compulsive disorder, substance abuse, and psy-
chosis), especially if the diagnosis of an eating disorder is not
totally clear. It should also be noted that, contrary to earlier opinion
several decades ago, all of the conditions listed in the differential
diagnosis can also be comorbid with an eating disorder, thus any
given patient can have both an eating disorder and another medical
or psychiatric condition. In fact, many patients with eating disorders do have other psychiatric conditions (which can both exacer-
bate or be exacerbated by the eating disorder).

The medical complications of eating disorders that do not vary
significantly by age include the following: (1) Metabolic abnormalities—most patients with anorexia nervosa have normal electrolytes [10–12]. Alternatively, patients who drink excessive
amounts of fluids, especially water (either to make the scale read
higher on check-ups and/or to satisfy hunger without the ingestion
of calories) may have hyponatremia. In contrast, some (but not
most) patients with bulimia nervosa will be found to have a hypo-
kalemic, hypochloremic, metabolic alkalosis (i.e., low potassium,
low chloride, high CO_2) due to vomiting and/or laxative/diuretic

use [13]. The hypokalemia can reach life-threatening levels, so it is important that practitioners obtain electrolytes on all patients with eating disorders, especially those suspected of having bulimia nervosa. (2) Cardiovascular abnormalities—Patients with anorexia nervosa who have significant weight loss will usually be found to have bradycardia and/or orthostatic hypotension. If these are significant, they serve as a cause for a medical hospitalization. Some patients with either AN or BN can have a prolonged QT interval, while patients with BN who have hypokalemia can have U waves on an electrocardiogram. (3) Gastrointestinal (GI) abnormalities—almost every patient with an eating disorder has GI symptoms at some point in the course of their illness. Patients with AN often have abdominal pains, usually due to constipation, either when they are not eating or when they start to eat again after a long period of poor intake. Patients with bulimia nervosa can have esophageal irritation, destruction of tooth enamel, and can see isolated blood with vomiting even though it is rare for patients to have an esophageal tear. (4) Neurologic abnormalities—patients who lose a significant amount of weight, especially if it is in a relatively short period of time, will show evidence of cerebral atrophy on a magnetic resonance imaging (MRI) scan [14]. It is thought that this resolves with refeeding. Rarely, patients with hyponatremia from excessive water intake can have seizures. Patients with a very large weight loss can develop a neuromyopathy, which generally resolves quickly with refeeding. (5) Hematologic abnormalities—ironically, the amenorrhea that develops in patients with anorexia nervosa generally protects these patients from developing anemia, so significant anemia is a rare finding in patients with eating disorders. Some patients with a major weight loss can develop neutropenia, and with an even greater loss, thrombocytopenia.

In anorexia nervosa, multiple alterations are seen in different endocrine axes as an adaption to the energy-deficient state. These include the following: (1) Thyroid abnormalities—patients with anorexia nervosa generally develop a relative hypothyroidism, as the body's way to conserve energy. This is mediated centrally, rendering T3, T4 and TSH low or low-normal. There is also the development of the euthyroid sick syndrome, whereby T3 tends to be even lower than T4. (2) Cortisol—in anorexia nervosa, the hypothalamic–pituitary–adrenal axis is stimulated, resulting in increased levels of cortisol. High cortisol levels have been shown to result in a decrease in the secretion of gondatropins, thereby contributing to the amenorrhea that is frequently seen in this population [15]. Additionally, increased cortisol levels also add to the problem of decreased bone mass through a variety of different mechanisms. (3) IGF-1/GH—GH stimulates secretion of IGF-1 and both are found to have anabolic properties on bone. Typically, both IGF-1 and GH are increased during puberty, a time of rapid growth and bone mass accrual. In individuals with anorexia nervosa, GH concentrations are found to be increased, likely related to reduced truncal fat [16]. Despite these increased GH concentrations, however, concentrations of IGF-1 are found to be low, suggesting resistance to GH. These aberrations in GH and IGF-1 further contribute to the impaired bone metabolism that is observed in anorexia nervosa. (4) Leptin/Ghrelin—leptin, an adiopokine involved in appetite suppression, may have a direct effect on the pulsatile secretion of GnRH. In patients with anorexia nervosa, leptin levels are low, likely as a protective mechanism. Leptin is believed to directly impact GnRH pulsation, affecting both amplitude and frequency, such that low levels of leptin can alter GnRH pulsations, inhibiting the hypothalamic–pituitary axis. Ghrelin, an appetite stimulating hormone and GH secretagogue, has also been found to be an inhibitor of gonadotropin secretion [17]. (5) LH/FSH/estradiol—In response to starvation, there is development of low levels of LH and FSH and long-term suppression of the hypothalamic–pituitary axis. Prior studies have indicated underdeveloped pulsations of LH in patients with anorexia nervosa, similar to patterns seen in the pre-pubertal or early pubertal stages of LH secretion [18]. Estradiol levels are also decreased. As a result of a prolonged hypoestrogenic state, long-term effects to bone mineral density are seen which are not fully reversible once weight gain is achieved, leading to the development of osteopenia and osteoporosis [19, 20].

The amenorrhea that occurs in patients with AN can be primary amenorrhea or it can be secondary amenorrhea. In cases of delayed menarche due to AN it is, of course, difficult to know when menarche would otherwise have occurred, unless the patient and/or family are able to indicate when thelarche had occurred. In the patient in the vignette it is likely she would not have had menarche by the time she initially presented at 11 years of age, especially since her mother indicated that many others in the family had a late onset of menarche. This may or may not have been due to the fact that the "women in the family tend to be thin." It is likely, however, that she should have had the onset of menarche at some point between 11 and 14 years of age and that the absence of menarche by this point is likely due to the on-going malnutrition, although even this cannot be said with certainty given her specific family history. In general, however, whether it is primary or secondary amenorrhea that is the issue for a particular patient with AN, a major goal of treatment is to achieve the weight gain that is necessary for the onset or return of menses for that patient.

The amount of weight that needs to be gained for the return of menses in those with secondary amenorrhea or for the onset of menses in delayed menarche/primary amenorrhea, however, is looked at differently in these two situations. In those with secondary amenorrhea, the older literature indicated that most patients needed to return to 90 % of average body weight for return of menses [21, 22]. While that remains true for many of the patients who start out at a normal weight and then lose enough weight to develop amenorrhea, that is usually not true for patients who start out overweight, become underweight, and develop amenorrhea along the way. These patients generally need to regain weight to an amount that is somewhere between their original starting weight and what would be the average weight for their height. It is not always possible to know exactly what that weight is for any individual patient, although in some cases the weight at which menses stopped may be used as a goal weight for the possible or likely return of menses. Hormonal therapy to induce menses is not recommended and emphasis should be placed on weight gain in order to achieve menses.

For patients with delayed menarche/primary amenorrhea, determining the amount of weight to be gained involves examining the patient's pattern of growth prior to the development of the eating disorder. In those patients, there is usually delayed growth that accompanies the weight loss and delayed menses. For instance, the patient's growth curve (Fig. 8.1) shows that she likely would have been approximately 110 lb and 63 in. at 14 years of age had she followed her curves (approximately the 50th percentile for both weight and height). Instead she is now 80 lb (the 3rd percentile for weight) and 61 in. (the 25th percentile for height). Thus she is approximately 30 lb and 2 in. less than she likely would have been had she not had an eating disorder. In a case such as this, it is a return to the normal growth curves that is often required for onset of menses. In accomplishing this, it is important that patients and parents understand that continuous weight gain is needed for this to happen and that the height will lag behind the weight (as opposed to height and weight increasing simultaneously in normal growth) during the treatment phase. This concept is particularly difficult for patients with eating disorders (and their families) because it means that there truly need to be points along the way where the patient may be somewhat "overweight" by classic definitions. It is very unlikely that this patient will begin menarche before she returns to the 50th percentile for weight. In addition, a return to the 50th percentile for weight is also likely to ultimately result in a return to the 50th percentile for height (or almost the 50th percentile for height, because there are some studies that indicate that patients who develop AN before completing their growth end up approximately ½ in. shorter than their adult height would have been) [23, 24]. A discussion of the effects of AN on adolescent growth and the achievement of full adult height is often all that is needed to get many pre- or peri-pubertal males with AN to reverse their weight loss, but this is less predictably useful for pre- and peri-pubertal girls, many of whom say, especially while the eating disorder is ongoing, that they do not care about whether they are potentially delaying their growth and stunting their height.

Since the adolescent years are the years in which peak bone mass is achieved, and since patients with amenorrhea due to nutritional causes (including those with the female athlete triad) lose bone mass while they are amenorrheic, the adolescents with amenorrhea, in essence, have a "double problem" (i.e., they are not increasing their bone density in the same way that they should and instead are losing bone density in the same way that adult women do following menopause). Multiple studies have shown that the only reliable treatment for the osteopenia/osteoporosis is a return to normal eating, normal weight, and normal menses [25, 26].

However, the bone density that was lost during the time of the amenorrhea is most likely not made up during the following years. It is thus crucial that a return to normal weight and menses be accomplished as quickly as possible in order to limit the damage to the bones as much as possible. Ultimately, the effects of the osteopenia/osteoporosis are not felt during the adolescent or young adult years (although some studies indicate there is an increased fracture risk during that time) but the major problem will likely occur when the patient who had an eating disorder enters her later adult years with a lower bone density than she should have had. In a study of bone density testing performed by dual energy X-ray absorptiometry (DXA) on 80 patients of ours with amenorrhea of at least 6–12 months, we found no patients with above average bone density for age (whereas half of the patients should have been above average), indicating that all of our patients lost bone density, and patients with greater than 2–2 ½ years of amenorrhea all had bone density levels in the "osteoporosis" range for age [27]. Studies have also shown that such treatments as vitamin D and calcium or birth control pills, or even bisphosphonates, do not ameliorate the bone density loss (although some recent studies have shown that physiologic doses of estrogen may be helpful in those with the most severe cases of AN) [26, 28]. It is therefore essential that patients return to normal weight and normal menses as quickly as possible. This is true both for those with delayed menarche/primary amenorrhea, as well as for those with secondary amenorrhea.

Management

Evaluation of patients with eating disorders includes determination of medical, nutritional, and psychological factors. Evaluation begins with performance of a complete history, with a focus on when and why dietary changes and other eating disorder behaviors began and how they proceeded and changed over time. In the adolescent patient, especially the younger adolescent patient, what steps the family has taken, both at home and in seeking outside help, are explored. As is standard for all medical histories, the past medical history, family history, and review of systems are obtained. Vital signs are obtained, either before or after the history is obtained, with weight, height, blood pressure, and pulse each being a crucial part of the evaluation. A complete physical examination is performed, looking for evidence of malnutrition, evaluating Tanner stages in the older child and younger adolescent, and searching for other abnormalities which could signify the presence of another underlying illness as part of the differential diagnosis. A nutrition history is performed, determining in detail what the patient has been eating and how that has changed over time; asking questions about binging and purging, use of diet pills, laxatives, diuretics, and/or supplements, and types and amounts of exercise; and finding out how the weight loss progressed over time and what weight the patient now says she would like to be [29].

Answers to these questions, especially in the presentation of the younger adolescent, are confirmed both by the parents verbally and with a growth chart, if available. The growth curves for weight and height (Fig. 8.1) should be utilized to follow the curve to see what the weight (and height) should be. The patient's growth curve shows that while her weight on first presentation at 11 years of age had fallen from 78 to 65 lb (a decrease of 13 lb, which is 18 %), in fact her weight should have been 82 lb at 11 years of age, so she was actually 17 lb (20 %) below where she should have been. An even larger difference is found at her 14-year-old visit. While her weight is 80 lb and her height is 61 in. at this point, putting her at 20–25 lb below the expected weight of 100–105 lb at her current height, in fact her growth curve shows that she should have been 110–115 lb and 63 in., putting her 30–35 lb below her expected weight (and 2 in. below her expected height) at this time. For the sake of this chapter, it is important to be aware of the effects of malnutrition on growth and to always attempt to get a growth curve going back to early childhood for any pre- or peri-pubertal patient being evaluated for anorexia nervosa.

Lastly, a psychosocial evaluation is performed. This includes questions about issues at home, in school, with friends and in outside activities; mental health symptoms, both in the past and more recently, that may indicate the presence of depression, anxiety, obsessive-compulsive traits or disorder, and other mental health conditions; a possible history of physical or emotional or sexual abuse; health risk behaviors, including smoking, drinking, drug use, and sexual activity; and a family history, both in the immediate family and also the more distant family, of mental health conditions, especially the presence of eating disorders. As we now are over 40 years into the eating disorder epidemic that began in the 1960s and 1970s, it is becoming increasingly more common for there to be a history of an eating disorder in the patient's mother, which has many implications for therapy.

As is true for evaluation, the treatment of patients with eating disorders involves medical, nutritional, and psychological components. These various aspects of treatment can take place in different settings, depending on the level of severity of the individual patient. For the mildest cases, treatment in the community by a pediatrician, nutritionist and therapist will often suffice to bring about the reversal in "mood and food and attitude" required for a return to normal eating, normal periods, normal mood, and a "normal" life. More severe cases may require a specialized eating disorder treatment center, mostly still in out-patient settings. The most severe cases, such as that described in the vignette, require a "higher level of care." This can take place in a day or evening program, a residential facility, or a hospitalization on a medical or psychiatric unit.

The medical and nutritional aspects of care are generally managed together. Electrolyte or cardiac abnormalities, such as hypokalemia or severe bradycardia (generally below 40 beats per minute) require immediate attention, usually in a hospital setting [30]. Other medical abnormalities generally resolve over time, as nutrition and weight improve, usually by increasing calorie intake 100–200 cal per day for those who are hospitalized or 400–600 cal per week for those who are out-patients. Care must be taken in those who are severely malnourished, especially those who have lost a large amount of weight relatively rapidly, to not cause the "refeeding syndrome." The refeeding syndrome was first described at the end of World War II when it observed in concentration camp survivors who were provided with nutrition too quickly following prolonged starvation [31]. A critical feature of the refeeding syndrome is the development of hypophosphatemia. Depletion of phosphorus occurs as increased insulin due to refeeding causes hormonal and metabolic changes to occur that require the use of adenosine triphosphate (ATP). The refeeding syndrome can result in the development of cardiac failure or hemolytic anemia and, most commonly, delirium or stupor or even coma. The refeeding syndrome can be ameliorated, and usually prevented, by use of slow refeeding in in-patient settings and the addition of phosphorus supplementation to the dietary plan. It is interesting to note that the patient in the vignette was not at risk for the refeeding syndrome because the problem for this patient, and other young patients like her, is failure to gain appropriate weight, rather than a significant weight loss per se. Thus, when the patient was admitted to the hospital, as she finally was on the follow-up visit described, calorie increases were able to be applied without the addition of supplemental phosphorus.

Almost all patients with eating disorders require formal psychological therapy along with the medical and nutritional aspects of care [29]. In earlier times, most patients received standard interpersonal therapy, but this was not always successful with adolescent patients, especially the younger adolescents who did not have the cognitive maturity to fully benefit from it. Over time, other types of therapy, better tailored to patients with eating disorders, have been developed. These include cognitive behavioral therapy (CBT), utilized for both younger and older adolescents, dialectical behavior therapy (DBT), most beneficial for those with more severe underlying psychopathology, and family-based therapy (FBT), referred to as the Maudsley approach after the hospital in England where it was developed, in which parents are given the skills to be able to get their children to eat the amounts they require and gain the amounts they need. In Adolescent Medicine settings, informal behavioral approaches are also utilized. Thus external "threats" such as not being able to participate in sports activities or school trips or being required to go to a "higher level of care" if increased nutrition or appropriate weight gain are not accomplished, may be able to provide needed motivation to move forward with the nutritional aspects of care. Ultimately, it is the combination of medical and nutritional care, along with formal and informal psychological approaches, that result in step by step improvements for most patients with anorexia nervosa. In some cases, pharmacotherapy, in the form of selective serotonin reuptake inhibitors (SSRIs), or occasionally the newer antipsychotic class of medications, are required adjuncts to care. However, it is clear in the medical literature that medication use is more effective for bulimia nervosa (sometimes resulting in a lowering in the urge to binge and/or purge) than it is in anorexia nervosa, and special care is used in giving these medications to younger patients because of a black box warning that the SSRIs can cause suicidal ideation and the antipsychiatric medications can cause cardiac effects. In addition, there are indications that SSRI medications do not work well, even for depression, in those who are severely underweight [32].

Finally, the literature indicates that the prognosis for patients with eating disorders is "guarded." Fifty percent of patients do well, 30 % do "okay," and 20 % do poorly. There is a 1 % mortality rate per year, 50 % of which is medical and 50 % of which is by suicide. These data generally come from studies in adults, and mostly from in-patient psychiatric settings [33, 34]. In contrast, the prognosis in adolescents, especially young adolescents, even those with a protracted course, is actually very good, with 75–85 % doing very well over time. It is for this reason that we encourage parents to be both optimistic in their outlook and aggressive in their treatment, and we reassure them that they will generally be rewarded with a good outcome, even if they must endure an arduous course.

Outcome

The patient was admitted to our hospital, where she succeeded in increasing from a 1200 cal per day diet on the day after admission to a 2600 cal per day diet 1 week later, when she was transferred to a psychiatric unit specializing in the treatment of eating disorders in young adolescents. She gained 4 lb during her week on our medical unit and an additional 14 lb during her 2 months in the psychiatric unit, from where she returned to resume out-patient care in a better frame of mind and more interested in gaining weight, growing, going on to achieve menarche, and returning to a normal life for girls her age.

Clinical Pearls/Pitfalls

1. Eating disorders, anorexia nervosa and related conditions, represent one of the major causes of abnormal female puberty.
2. The changes made in the DSM-5 for the diagnosis of eating disorders have been very helpful in establishing criteria that more accurately reflect the most appropriate diagnoses in children and peri-pubertal adolescents.
3. The medical complications of eating disorders occur similarly in all age groups, but primary amenorrhea and delays in growth and development are specific to peri-pubertal adolescents.
4. Females affected by anorexia nervosa develop long-term suppression of the hypothalamic–pituitary axis, which can result in long term effects on bone mineral density.
5. Examination of the prior growth pattern through the use of growth curves is a useful tool to determine the amount of weight to be gained for patients with an eating disorder and delayed menarche.
6. The treatment of patients with eating disorders involves a multidisciplinary approach including medical, nutritional, and psychological components.
7. Hormonal therapy to induce or regulate the menstrual cycle is not recommended. Emphasis should be placed on weight gain and organized adequate caloric intake in order to achieve menarche or normalize the menstrual cycle for girls with eating disorders.

References

1. Golden NH, Katzman DK, Kreipe RE, et al. Eating disorders in adolescents: Position paper of the society for adolescent medicine. J Adolesc Health. 2003;33:496–503.
2. American Academy of Pediatrics, Committee on Adolescence. Clinical report-identification and management of eating disorders in children and adolescents. Pediatrics. 2010;126:1240–1253.
3. American Psychiatric Association. Diagnostic and Statistical Manual of Mental Disorders. 4th ed. Arlington: American Psychiatric Association; 1994.
4. American Psychiatric Association. Diagnostic and statistical manual of mental disorders. 5th ed. Arlington: American Psychiatric Association; 2013.

5. Fisher M, Gonzalez, Malizio J. Eating disorders in adolescents. How does the DSM-5 change the diagnosis? Int J Adolesc Med Health. 2015;27(4):437–41.
6. Golden NH, Carlson JL. The pathophysiology of amenorrhea in the adolescent. Ann N Y Acad Sci. 2008;1135:163–78.
7. Drewnowski A, Hopkins AS, Kessler RC. The prevalence of bulimia nervosa in the US college student population. Am J Public Health. 1998;78(10):1322–5.
8. Szabo P, Tury F. The prevalence of bulimia nervosa in a Hungarian college and secondary school population. Psychother Psychosom. 1999;56:43–7.
9. Fisher MM, Rosen DS, Ornstein RM, Mammel KA, Katzman DK, Rome ES, Callahan ST, Malizio J, Kearny S, Walsh BT. Characteristics of avoidant/restrictive food intake disorder in children and adolescents: a "new disorder in DSM-5. J Adolesc Health. 2014;55(1):49–52.
10. Fisher M. Medical complications of anorexia and bulimia nervosa. Adolesc Med State Art Rev. 1992;3:487–502.
11. Palla B, Litt IF. Medical complications of eating disorders in adolescents. Pediatrics. 1998;81:613–23.
12. Katzman DK. Medical complications in adolescents with anorexia nervosa: A review of the literature. Int J Eat Disord. 2005;37(Suppl):52–9.
13. Golden NH. Eating disorders in adolescence and their sequelae. Best Pract Res Clin Obstet Gynaecol. 2003;17:57–73.
14. Kingston K, Szmukler G, Andrewes D, Tress B, Desmond P. Neuropsychological and structural brain changes in anorexia nervosa before and after refeeding. Psychol Med. 1996;26:15–28.
15. Misra M, Arabhakaran R, Miller KK, et al. Role of cortisol in the menstrual recovery in adolescent girls with anorexia nervosa. Pediatr Res. 2006;59:588–603.
16. Misra M, Miller KK, Almazan C, Worley M, Herzog DB, Klibanski A. Hormonal determinants of regional body composition in adolescent girls with anorexia nervosa and control. J Clin Endocrinol Metab. 2005;90:2580–7.
17. Kojima M, Hosoda H, Date Y, et al. Ghrelin is a growth-hormone releasing acylated peptide from stomach. Nature. 1999;402:656–60.
18. Singhal V, Misra M, Klibanski A. Endocrinology of anorexia nervosa in young people: recent insights. Curr Opin Endocrinol Diabetes Obes. 2014;21:64–70.
19. Bacharah LK, Guido D, Katzman D, et al. Decreased bone density in adolescent girls with anorexia nervosa. Pediatrics. 1990;86:440–7.
20. Katzman D, Zipursky R. Adolescents with anorexia nervosa: the impact of the disorder on bones and brains. Ann N Y Acad Sci. 1990;817:127–37.
21. Frisch RE, McArthur JW. Menstrual cycles: Fatness as a determinant of minimum weight for height necessary for their maintenance or onset. Science. 1974;185:949.
22. Golden NH, Jacobson MS, Schebendach J, Palestro CJ, Jacobson MS, Shenker IR. Resumption of menses in anorexia nervosa. Arch Pediatr Adolesc Med. 1997;151:16–21.

23. Danzinger Y, Maukamei M, Zeharia A, Dinari G, Mimouni M. Stunting of growth in anorexia nervosa during the prepubertal period. Isr J Med Sci. 1994;30:581–4.
24. Lantzouni E, Frank GR, Golden NH, Shenker RI. Reversibility of growth stunting in early onset anorexia: a prospective study. J Adolesc Health. 2002;31:162–5.
25. Golden NH, Jacobson MS, Schebendach J, Solanto MV, Hertz SM, Shenker IR. Resumption of menses in anorexia nervosa. Arch Pediatr Adolesc Med. 2002;151:16–21.
26. Golden NH. Osteopenia and osteoporosis in anorexia nervosa. Adolesc Med State Art Rev. 2003;14:97–108.
27. Schneider M, Fisher M, Wienerman S, Lesser M. Correlates of low bone density in females with anorexia nervosa. Int J Adolosc Med Health. 2002;14:297–306.
28. Golden NH, Iglesias EA, Jacobson MS, Carey D, Meyer W, Schebendach J, et al. Alendronate for the treatment of osteopenia in anorexia nervosa. A randomized double-blind, placebo-controlled trial. J Clin Endocrinol Metabol. 2005;90:3179–85.
29. Lock J, Via MC. American Academy of Child and Adolescent Psychiatry Committee on Quality Issues. Practice parameter for the assessment and treatment of children and adolescents with eating disorders. J Am Acad Child Adolesc Psychiatry. 2015;54:412–25.
30. Golden NH, Katzman DK, Sawyer SM, Ornstein RM, Rome ES, Garber AK, Kohn M, Kreipe RE. Position Paper of the Society for Adolescent Health and Medicine: Medical management of restrictive eating disorders in adolescents and young adults. J Adolesc Health. 2015;56:121–5.
31. Brozek J, Chapman C, Keys A. Drastic food restriction: effects on cardio-vascular dynamics in normotensive and hypertensive conditions. JAMA. 1948;137:1569–74.
32. Attia E, Haiman C, Walsh BT, Flater SR. Does fluoxetine augment the inpatient treatment of anorexia nervosa? Am J Psychiatry. 2008;155:548–51.
33. Fisher M. The course and outcome of eating disorders in adults and in adolescents: A review. Adolesc Med State Art Rev. 2003;14:149–58.
34. Steinhausen H-C. The outcome of anorexia nervosa in the 20th century. Am J Psychiatry. 2002;159:1284–93.

Chapter 9
The Female Athlete Triad and Abnormal Pubertal Development

Maria C. Monge

Abbreviations

ACSM	American College of Sports Medicine
BMD	Bone mineral density
BMI	Body mass index
COC	Combination oral contraceptive
DHEA-S	Dehydroepiandrosterone sulfate
DSM-5	Diagnostic and Statistical Manual of Mental Disorders: 5th edn
DXA	Dual-energy X-ray absorptiometry
FFM	Fat free mass
FSH	Follicle-stimulating hormone
GnRH	Gonadotropin releasing hormone
HCG	Human chorionic gonadotropin
IGF-1	Insulin-like growth factor 1

M.C. Monge, M.D. (✉)
Dell Children's Medical Center of Central Texas, University
of Texas at Austin, Dell Medical School, 4900 Mueller Blvd,
Austin, TX 78723, USA
e-mail: maria.c.monge@gmail.com; mmonge@utexas.edu

© Springer International Publishing Switzerland 2016
H.L. Appelbaum (ed.), *Abnormal Female Puberty*,
DOI 10.1007/978-3-319-27225-2_9

LH	Luteinizing hormone
NCAA	National Collegiate Athletic Association
PPE	Pre-participation physical examination
T3	Triiodothyronine
T4	Thyroxine
Triad	Female athlete triad
TSH	Thyroid stimulating hormone

Case Presentation

A 16-year-old girl is brought to the office by her mother for evaluation of secondary amenorrhea. She is previously healthy and is an avid, multi-sport athlete, playing soccer, cross-country and track. She has never had any serious medical problems and does not take any medications. Last fall she had to miss the entire cross-country season due to a metatarsal stress fracture that was diagnosed early in preseason training.

Menarche was at age 11 and after an initial few months of irregularity, her cycle length was fairly consistent at 28–29 days. Over the last year, her periods became irregular again and her last menstrual period was 8 months ago. In confidential history, she denies being sexually active. Her review of systems is negative other than occasional headaches. She had a 15 lb intentional weight loss 9 months ago, but since her weight has been stable. She says that her current weight is good for all of her sports where speed is important. She eats three small meals per day and occasionally has an afternoon snack. She currently exercises 2–3 h per day. She adamantly denies any self-induced vomiting or use of diet pills, laxatives or diuretics. Her Eating Attitudes Test [1] was not suggestive of an eating disorder.

On physical examination her BMI is 18.4 (90.2 % of median BMI for her age). Her resting supine heart rate is 56 and blood pressure is 104/70. She is not orthostatic. She has mild facial acne but no hirsutism. She has no other skin lesions. She has Tanner 5 breast and pubic hair development. Her cardiac exam is notable for slight bradycardia, but is otherwise normal. She has no bony tenderness or musculoskeletal abnormalities.

Laboratory testing showed normal levels of prolactin, follicle-stimulating hormone (FSH), testosterone, and dehydroepiandrosterone-sulfate (DHEA-S), but luteinizing hormone (LH) was slightly low. Urine human chorionic gonadotropin (hCG) was negative. Thyroid testing was notable for a low free triiodothyronine (T3) with normal thyroid stimulating hormone (TSH) and free thyroxine (T4). Estradiol level was undetectable. Bone mineral density was tested using dual-energy X-ray absorptiometry (DXA) and was low with Z-scores at lumbar spine and total body -1.8 and -1.7, respectively.

From this information the patient was diagnosed with functional hypothalamic amenorrhea as a consequence of the female athlete triad.

Discussion

Regular physical activity has numerous benefits in the overall health of an adolescent female including improved strength and endurance, reduced anxiety and stress, increased self-esteem, better school performance, and less risk-taking behavior [2, 3] and in the United States, the current recommendation for physical activity in adolescents is 60 min per day [2]. However, for many years, it has been recognized that in some females, exercise can lead to adverse health consequences. In 1992, a clinical syndrome entitled the female athlete triad (Triad) was described by a panel of experts convened by the American College of Sports Medicine (ACSM) and was described as an association of disordered eating, amenorrhea, and osteoporosis seen in activities that emphasized lean physique [4, 5]. This led to the ACSM issuing a position stand on the Triad in 1997, which further described this association [6]. Ongoing research in the area resulted in an updated position stand in 2007 which referred to three interrelated spectrums of energy availability, menstrual function, and bone mineral density and is now the accepted model for the Triad [7]. This model emphasizes that all exercising females are at risk for complications of the Triad and not just those with an eating disorder, although risk is highest in adolescents participating in sports emphasizing leanness [7].

Components of the Triad (Fig. 9.1)

Energy availability: Energy availability in exercising adolescent females is defined as the amount of dietary energy intake (kcal/day) minus the amount of energy expended in exercise (kcal/day) [8]. The amount of energy remaining is the energy available to complete the body's physiologic processes including such things as metabolic function, growth, and reproduction. Optimal energy availability for a normal weight, healthy young female athlete is approximately 45 kcal/kg FFM/day [8] and detrimental physiologic changes in reproductive function, bone health, and general metabolic processes occur at less than 30 kcal/kg FFM/day [9]. Low

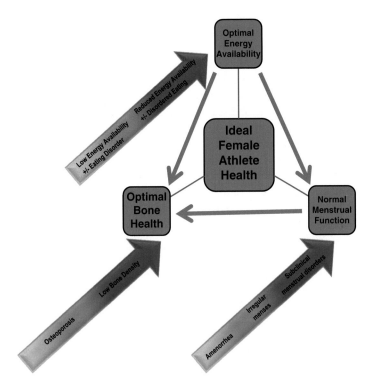

Fig. 9.1 Components of female athlete triad

energy availability does not occur exclusively in girls who are underweight, thus recognition of risk factors for this component of the Triad is important in identification.

Athletes who have low energy availability can arrive at this state through three mechanisms [7]. First, an athlete may be inadvertently eating too few calories to sustain the current level of exercise, which can be especially problematic when training and competition intensity are high, such as mid-season [10]. Female athletes in this category may not have obvious signs of low energy availability such as weight loss, as total body energy balance can remain stable (i.e., weight maintenance) while energy availability is low [7, 11]. In these cases, deficits in energy availability may only be detected by signs of chronic energy deficiency such as low resting metabolic rate [12, 13] or low T3 [9, 12, 13] or through health consequences such as menstrual disturbances.

Next, an athlete may be purposefully altering energy availability to try to improve performance and/or change body composition by either increasing energy expended during exercise and not increasing energy intake or by decreasing energy intake while exercise energy expenditure remains constant [7]. These athletes may exhibit disordered eating behaviors without meeting criteria for an eating disorder but may employ unhealthy weight modification techniques such as fasting, purging, laxative use and diet pill use [7]. Typically, these athletes have evidence of recent weight decline or changes in body fat composition.

Finally, some athletes meet DSM-5 criteria [14] for eating disorders such as anorexia nervosa, atypical anorexia nervosa, or bulimia nervosa and have low energy availability due to their eating disorder as well as their ongoing energy expenditure from exercise [15] and some studies suggest that the prevalence of eating disorders is higher in athletes than in non-athletes [16, 17]. Sports emphasizing leanness or physique have a higher prevalence of eating disorders among their athletes [18].

Anorexia nervosa is defined by restrictive eating resulting in a significantly low body weight as the result of an intense fear of weight gain and disturbance in the way weight or shape is experienced which is often accompanied by denial of the seriousness of the low weight. Amenorrhea is no longer a criteria used in diagnosing anorexia nervosa. In atypical anorexia nervosa, patients have all of the features of anorexia nervosa, but their body weight is in the normal range. Bulimia nervosa is an eating disorder in which a patient has repeated cycles (at least once per week for 3 months) of binge eating followed by compensatory behaviors such as self-induced vomiting, use of laxatives or diuretics, fasting, or excessive exercise. Similar to patients with anorexia nervosa, patients with bulimia nervosa have self-perceptions that are unduly influenced by their weight and shape [14]. Athletes who have low energy availability due to an eating disorder may present with low body weight or attitudes and behaviors concerning for an eating disorder; however, others may go undetected unless questioned. Because tools for measuring energy expenditure as well as energy intake (including dietary logs) can be impractical [10] and imprecise [19, 20], it has been recommended that all athletes at risk for low energy availability undergo evaluation by a sports dietician [21].

Menstrual function: Regular monthly menses are an indicator of overall health status in adolescent females and there is significant evidence that intense athletic training in adolescents, especially when accompanied by undernutrition, can lead to menstrual abnormalities [22–24]. Young gymnasts and ballet dancers often have delayed menarche by 2–3 years as compared to family members and irregular menses and secondary amenorrhea are common findings in these girls [22–25]. In a 2003 study by Beals, 22.2 % of girls in aesthetic sports had not had a period by the age of 16 [26] versus 1 % of the general population [27]. Menstrual abnormalities in exercising females can be thought of on a spectrum from eumenorrhea (regular ovulatory monthly menstrual cycles) to amenorrhea [7] with prevalence estimates of primary and secondary amenorrhea being 0–56 % and 1–60.0 %, respectively [15]. Subtle menstrual disorders such as luteal phase defects and anovulation may not be clinically detectable as menstrual cycles remain perceptibly normal, but these disorders are very common in exercising females [28] with estimated prevalence ranging from 5.9 to 43.0 % [15] versus sedentary women with prevalence of around 5 % [28].

   Disruption of menstrual function in exercising females is not due to the direct effects of the exercise [29] but instead is a "functional" adaptation from low energy availability as reproductive function is suppressed as a strategy to prevent pregnancy and further energy expenditure [30]. This is an important distinction as there is often a common misperception that menstrual disturbance in exercising adolescents is "normal" and thus no further evaluation is needed.

Functional hypothalamic amenorrhea results from a decrease in pulsatile release of GnRH from the hypothalamus, which in turn leads to a decrease in pulsatile release of gonadotropins from the pituitary gland and subsequent menstrual disturbance with decreased levels of circulating estrogen [30]. Regulation of the hypothalamic release of GnRH is not completely understood, though leptin, a hormone secreted by adipose tissue that plays a role in appetite regulation and energy expenditure [31], is thought to play a role [32], with relative changes in leptin levels possibly being more important than absolute levels [33]. Disruption in LH pulsatility occurs quickly once energy availability drops below 30 kcal/kg FFM/day and changes in LH levels can be measured as early as 5 days [9], demonstrating the very sensitive nature of this system to adequate energy availability.

Bone health: Although bone health is an issue that, more typically, is addressed in adulthood, bone mass that is achieved in the child and adolescent years is thought to be the most important modifiable determinant of lifelong skeletal health [34]. Bone accrual primarily occurs in the first two decades of life with 90 % of bone mass achieved by the age of 18 [35]. There are many factors that contribute to overall bone health including genetics, gender and ethnicity, all considered non-modifiable factors, as well as nutritional status, exercise, body weight and composition and hormonal status, which are considered modifiable factors [36].

The skeleton is a dynamic organ undergoing continuous remodeling and there are multiple circulating factors that contribute to its health including cytokines, estrogen, parathyroid hormone, 1,25-dihydroxyvitamin D, insulin-like growth factor-1 (IGF-1), and calcitonin [36], and alterations in any of these circulating factors can impact overall bone health. Energy availability also plays a direct role in bone health as bone trophic hormones require adequate energy availability for production [7]. Weight-bearing exercise generates mechanical loading forces on the skeleton and increases bone mass accrual in adolescents [37] and menstruating female adolescent athletes in weight-bearing sports have higher bone mineral density than non-athletes [36, 38, 39], although effects are more pronounced in sports with highest mechanical loading on the skeleton [23, 40]. Site-specific gains in bone mineral density are possible in certain sports depending on the mechanical loading pattern [36]. Bone mass accrual is not affected by participation in non-weight-bearing sports, such as swimming, water polo, or cycling [41].

In female adolescents, there is an especially pronounced effect of estrogen on bone health, as estrogen acts in a number of ways to inhibit bone resorption and regulate bone formation [42]. Continuous estrogen exposure from prepuberty through time of peak bone mass assures optimal accrual, thus adolescents with estrogen deficiency, such as those with menstrual disorders or those with delayed puberty, achieve lower peak bone mass [43, 44]. By extension, exercising adolescents with menstrual disorders would be expected to have lower peak bone mass [32]. Estrogen deficiency mitigates much of the effect of weight-bearing exercise on bone accrual, especially at trabecular bone sites where mechanical loads are lowest [32]. Female athletes with amenorrhea have lower bone mineral density at the spine and whole body compared to those who are eumenorrheic even with similar lean body mass [40]. There appears to be a dose–response relationship between energy availability and markers of bone turnover in exercising females [45] and bone turnover markers are lower in athletes with amenorrhea [40]. Distance runners seem to be at especially high risk for inadequate bone mass accrual as a cross-sectional study of female adolescent runners showed no significant difference in bone mineral content between runners ages 13–14 and 17–18, which was in contrast to non-runners who had normal increase in bone mineral content with age [46]. Additionally, as the number of risk factors for the Triad increases, there is a greater risk of low bone mineral density [47]. Concerted efforts should be made for early identification of female adolescent athletes who are at risk for low peak bone mass, as even with increased energy availability, weight gain, and resumption of normal menses, there seems to be incomplete catch-up of bone mass [23, 48, 49].

Adverse Health Consequences of the Triad

Adolescent females with one or more components of the Triad are at risk for adverse health outcomes, some of immediate health consequence and others with longer-term implications. These impacts can be on physical health as well as psychological health. An obvious consequence of menstrual disturbances is impaired reproductive function, which may be clearly identified in the cases of amenorrhea, but less obvious in cases of anovulation or luteal phase defects [7]. An increased risk for osteoporosis with resultant health complications is also a clear consequence of the Triad [7]. These areas of adverse health consequence as the result of the Triad may not be as obvious and deserve more attention.

Stress fractures and musculoskeletal injury: A stress fracture occurs when repetitive stress on a bone exceeds that bone's capacity to withstand and heal from those forces. Stress fracture risk seems to be linked to lower bone mass and menstrual irregularity [7, 50] and multiple studies have shown an increased risk of stress fracture in females with menstrual irregularity [47, 50–54]. Furthermore, exercising females who suffer from stress fracture, who have irregular or absent menses, seem to show higher grades of stress fracture on MRI than those with regular menses [55]. Other musculoskeletal injuries such as ligament sprains and muscle or tendon strains may also be more common in girls with components of the Triad as female high school athletes with disordered eating behaviors, low bone mineral density at the spine, and/or menstrual dysfunction all had increased risk of musculoskeletal injury [47]. Because much of the health risk associated with the Triad is perceived to be more long term, it may be difficult to attain "buy-in" from the adolescent athlete based on these risks alone. Therefore, the more immediate possibility of season or career-threatening injury (such as can happen with stress fracture or muscle, tendon, or ligament injury) can be of utmost importance when counseling girls on the importance of treating components of the Triad.

Endothelial dysfunction: The development of cardiovascular disease is a complex process; however, one of the known precipitants is endothelial cell dysfunction [3], especially in the coronary arteries.

Currently, the gold standard noninvasive method of measuring endothelial cell function is brachial artery ultrasonography to measure flow-mediated arterial dilation [56]. This measurement is then used as a proxy for coronary endothelial function which has been shown to predict cardiovascular health outcomes [3]. Recently, it has been discovered that in exercising females with low circulating estrogen, endothelial function seems to be impaired with subsequent implications for long-term cardiovascular health and retrospective data in these women suggest an increase in premature coronary artery disease [57]. The underlying mechanism of these effects involves decreased production of nitric oxide due to low estrogen levels (via nitric oxide synthatase) and thus decreased nitric oxide effects in blood vessels with less smooth muscle relaxation, as well as fewer anti-atherosclerotic effects [48, 58]. In two studies of female endurance athletes, those with amenorrhea had impaired endothelial function versus the other athletes in the studies [59, 60]. In another study of professional ballet dancers, over 60 % of the females in the study had impaired endothelial function and of those women the majority had menstrual dysfunction [61]. In addition to the long-term cardiovascular health implications of endothelial dysfunction, there may be more immediate sports performance effects in these athletes as decreased flow-mediated dilation can decrease blood flow to exercising muscle thereby decreasing maximum exercise tolerance [58].

Psychological impact: The psychological impact of disordered eating and diagnosed eating disorders can be striking. Comorbid diagnoses of anxiety and depression are common in patients with anorexia nervosa and bulimia nervosa [62] and rates of suicidal thoughts and completed suicide in these patients are among the highest of all mental disorders [63, 64]. Furthermore, less than half of patients with anorexia nervosa will fully recover and 20 % remain chronically affected [65] with mortality in these patients sixfold higher than age-matched individuals [66]. In addition to the athletes with eating disorders, girls who have suffered injuries, possibly due to Triad-related factors, may be at higher risk for anxiety and depression, especially during their recovery [67].

Management

Awareness of Triad components is important in diagnosis as an athlete with one component of the Triad should be assessed for all [7], keeping in mind that due to the interrelatedness of all three components of the triad (low energy availability, amenorrhea, osteoporosis), meeting criteria for all three is not necessary to suffer consequences.

History: A standard medical history should be obtained in all adolescents being evaluated for the Triad, but in addition, they should have a comprehensive history focused on each component. First, a detailed diet and exercise history should be obtained. This can include recent weight changes, attitude toward current weight, past or present dieting behaviors, a brief recall of dietary intake over the past 24 h as well as current exercise patterns with types of exercise. Collateral history from parents, coaches, and teammates may also be important [68]. Next, a menstrual history should be obtained including age at menarche and menstrual pattern over the past 6–12 months. Finally, an athlete's history of prior musculoskeletal injury including fractures, stress fractures, sprains, and strains should be elicited.

Physical exam: A thorough physical exam should be performed on all athletes suspected of having any component of the Triad [7]. This exam should include measurement of height, weight, and calculation of BMI with plotting on appropriate growth curves [68] to determine current growth parameters. Prior growth charts can be helpful in determining weight trends. Vital signs should be checked including measurement of heart rate, orthostatic blood pressure, and temperature as bradycardia, orthostatic hypotension, and hypothermia can be seen in athletes with Triad components [7]. Other physical signs of low energy availability may include lanugo and cold distal extremities while physical signs of self-induced vomiting can include parotid gland hypertrophy and abrasions or callouses on fingers [68]. If an athlete has a history of irregular or absent menses, attention should be paid to signs that could explain other etiologies of the menstrual dysfunction such as thyroid enlargement or acne, hirsutism, or clitoromegaly which could suggest androgen excess. Any girl presenting with primary amenorrhea should have a genital exam as it may be abnormal in up to 15 % of these patients (such as an absent or blind vagina or transverse vaginal septum) [69]; however, the genital exam in girls with the Triad is typically normal. A musculoskeletal exam including gait assessment may reveal occult injury that was not discovered on history.

Formal evaluation of energy availability: If a female athlete's initial screening, history, and/or physical exam is suggestive of any component of the Triad, further investigation should be pursued [58]. When measuring energy availability, the gold standard is a 72-h dietary record in conjunction with a 72-h exercise record or measurement from an accelerometer in attempt to quantify energy intake and expenditure [70]. Unfortunately, its reliability is largely determined by athlete participation and compliance, but outside of research settings, at this time there is no better alternative. Calculation of optimal energy availability for an individual athlete requires measurement of percent body fat, which can be obtained through a number of methods, with varying reliability and accessibility, including use of skin calipers, bioelectrical impedance, hydrostatic weighing, DXA, or air displacement plethysmography. The measured percent body fat is used to calculate fat-free mass by subtracting calculated fat mass from total body mass [FFM = Total body mass − (total body mass × % body fat/100)].

Eating attitudes and patterns can be explored further using a specific eating disorder screening tool such as the Eating Attitudes Test [1] or the Eating Disorder Examination Questionnaire [71]. If these additional screening tests suggest an eating disorder, such as anorexia nervosa, atypical anorexia nervosa, or bulimia nervosa, the athlete should be formally evaluated by a mental health professional as soon as possible. It is important to remember that diagnosis of an eating disorder is not necessary for an adolescent to have consequences of the Triad, thus any abnormality identified in evaluation of energy availability should be considered on the spectrum of Triad components for that athlete.

If an athlete meets criteria for an eating disorder, laboratory studies including complete blood count, electrolytes, calcium, magnesium, glucose, liver function testing, urinalysis, and thyroid testing including a free T3 should be obtained [68]. If there is uncertainty about the diagnosis, an erythrocyte sedimentation rate and a celiac screen can also be considered [68]. Athletes with low energy availability with or without disordered eating, who do not meet the criteria for an eating disorder, can have a similar laboratory investigation performed, but it is not essential. An electrocardiogram should be obtained in any athlete with cardiovascular signs or symptoms, electrolyte derangements, purging behaviors, or significant weight loss [68]. Overall, most laboratory results will be normal in athletes with low energy availability but normal results do not exclude serious illness or medical instability [68].

Formal evaluation of menstrual abnormalities: With respect to evaluation of menstrual abnormalities, the diagnosis of functional hypothalamic amenorrhea in exercising adolescent females is a diagnosis of exclusion, thus those athletes who present with primary or secondary amenorrhea should have laboratory testing to exclude other etiologies of menstrual abnormality [20]. Irregular menses should also be evaluated similarly and not immediately presumed to be due to hypothalamic disruption. Urine hCG to exclude pregnancy should be obtained in all girls. Additionally, levels of FSH, TSH, and prolactin should be examined to exclude premature ovarian insufficiency, prolactin-secreting tumor, and thyroid disease, respectively [69]. In girls who have signs of androgen excess, testosterone, DHEA-S, and early morning 17-hydroxyprogesterone should also be included in this evaluation to exclude polycystic ovarian syndrome, androgen-secreting tumors, and congenital adrenal hyperplasia [7]. Serum estradiol level can be obtained [7], although caution should be used in interpreting the value as levels can fluctuate throughout the day and the level should not be relied upon as the sole marker of estrogen sufficiency. A progesterone challenge (10 mg of oral medroxyprogesterone acetate daily for 7–10 days) can be administered to assess for withdrawal bleeding and is an indirect way to measure serum estrogen level as hypoestrogenic women should not have withdrawal bleeding. In an athlete who has functional hypothalamic amenorrhea, but has improved energy availability, and is nearing menstrual recovery, a withdrawal bleed may occur [7]. Formal evaluation for subclinical menstrual disturbances (luteal phase defects, anovulation) is not routinely done outside of the research setting. Low to normal gonadotropin levels and low estradiol level are classic findings in athletes with functional hypothalamic amenorrhea or menstrual irregularity due to low energy availability; however, these values may be normal. Thus, once other etiologies have been excluded, one can diagnose the athlete with menstrual irregularity secondary to Triad factors.

Formal evaluation of bone health: The assessment of bone health is less straightforward given that fracture risk depends not only on skeletal components such as bone mass, size, and geometry, but also on age, body weight, prior fracture history as well as type and force of injury [36]. However, because approximately 70 % of bone strength is determined by bone mass, it is often used as a surrogate marker for bone health, although decreased bone mass does not necessarily correspond to an increase in fracture risk in adolescents [36]. Bone mass is determined by Dual-energy X-ray absorptiometry (DXA) which calculates bone mineral density (BMD). There are known problems with the use of DXA, such as it being a two-dimensional measurement only and cannot account for bone depth or size [48]; however, it is the most widely available tool and uses low amounts of radiation in comparison to other techniques [72].

Although DXA is widely used to assess bone health, there is a lack of high quality evidence to support recommendations for DXA in adolescents [73]. Currently, guidelines recommend that DXA be obtained when a patient presents with evidence of a systemic disease or disorder that has been associated with increased fracture risk (such as chronic malnutrition, cystic fibrosis, eating disorders, hypogonadism, chronic glucocorticoid exposure, and osteogenesis imperfecta) and prior to initiation of any treatment directly targeting bone activity [73, 74]. These recommendations do not specifically address adolescent female athletes with components of the Triad. Because poor bone health often has no clinical signs or symptoms, it is important to know who to screen. However, it is not feasible for all exercising adolescent females to undergo DXA; therefore, the ACSM and Female Athlete Triad coalition have made recommendations for obtaining DXA based on an individual athlete's risk factors and clinical presentation and in general, recommend screening adolescent athletes with a cumulative history of hypoestrogenism or disordered eating/eating disorder for 6 or more months and/or a history of stress or minimal impact fracture [30] (Table 9.1). If Triad risk factors persist, repeat DXA should be obtained every 12 months, preferably on the same machine [20, 75].

The interpretation of DXA results is different in adolescents than in older adult women. Often, both T-scores and Z-scores are listed on a DXA report; however, in adolescents only the Z-score (the number of standard deviations above/below the age-matched mean) should be used to interpret BMD as it is a comparison to

Table 9.1 Considerations for obtaining DXA in exercising adolescent females

• ≥1 High-risk factors	
Or	
• ≥2 Moderate-risk factors	
Or	
• ≥1 Non-peripheral or ≥2 peripheral long bone traumatic fracture with 1+ high- or moderate-risk factor	
Or	
• ≥6 Months use of medication that may impact bone	

High-risk factors	Moderate-risk factors
Current or prior diagnosis of Eating Disorder	Current or prior history of disordered eating for 6+ months
Currently severely underweight:	Currently underweight:
BMI ≤17.5 kg/m²	BMI between 17.5 and 18.5 kg/m²
<85 % median BMI for age	85–95 % median BMI for age
Recent weight loss >10 % in 1 month	Recent weight loss 5–10 % in 1 month

(continued)

Table 9.1 (continued)

Menarche ≥16 years	Menarche 15–16 years
	Current irregular menses
	6–8 menses in past 12 months
Prior bony injury:	Prior bony injury:
2 Prior stress reactions/ fractures	1 Stress reaction/fracture
1 High-risk stress fracture	
1 Low energy non-traumatic fracture	
Prior DXA Z-score less than −2.0	Prior DXA Z-score between −1.0 and −2.0

Adapted from Joy E, De Souza MJ, Nattiv A, Misra M, Williams NI, Mallinson RJ, et al. 2014 female athlete triad coalition consensus statement on treatment and return to play of the female athlete triad. Curr. Sports Med. Rep. 13:219–32

age- and sex-matched peers [75]. The term "osteopenia" should not be used in adolescents and instead "low bone mass for age" should be used to indicate that Z-scores are low [74, 75]. The diagnosis of osteoporosis in adolescents is not made based on DXA alone (Z-score less than −2.0, as in postmenopausal females) but instead is made with either ≥1 vertebral compression fracture in the absence of local disease or high energy trauma or low BMD with Z-score less than or equal to −2.0 and fracture following mild to moderate trauma of either ≥2 long bones by the age of 10 or ≥3 long bones by the age of 19 [73].

Because female athletes in weight-bearing sports should have 5–15 % higher BMD than age-matched peers [38, 39], the ACSM recommends more stringent guidelines for diagnosis of low bone density in these athletes and Z-score less than −1.0 should be considered abnormal [7].

Treatment: The cornerstone of treatment for adolescents with Triad components is restoration of optimal energy availability, which can be achieved through increasing energy intake, decreasing energy expenditure, or a combination of the two [20]. A multidisciplinary treatment team involving the athlete, coach, athletic trainer, health care professional, dietician, and if needed, mental health professional should be the gold standard of any treatment regimen [7, 20, 58]. Any treatment plan needs to consider goals of the athlete in addition to goals of the treatment team as alliance building for better health and ultimate performance is a key component for success. Athletes may have specific training and competition goals that are different at various times throughout the year, depending on competition schedules, and thus a treatment plan mid-season may look different than a treatment plan in the off-season. For example, an athlete may be more willing to increase energy intake during the season as opposed to decreasing energy expenditure, which should be reflected in the treatment plan [20]. A systematic process to monitor progress and adherence to the plan should also be implemented including regular monitoring of the athlete by members of the treatment team and consideration of written contracts [20].

Non-pharmacologic interventions in the treatment of female adolescents with the triad center around increasing energy availability and depending on the underlying reason for low energy availability, treatment can be different. If an athlete has inadvertent undereating as the cause for the energy mismatch, meeting with a sports dietician for an evaluation of overall energy expenditure and energy intake with a plan focused on increasing energy availability may be sufficient to correct the imbalance [20]. If, however, there is a component of disordered eating, intentional weight loss, or a diagnosed eating disorder, nutritional counseling with a sports dietician alone is unlikely to be successful [7, 58]. Gradual dietary changes are most acceptable by athletes, often requiring months to achieve a target caloric intake. Ultimately, the target energy availability for adolescent athletes should be ≥45 kcal/kg FFM/day [20].

Counseling on nutritional requirements should also include addressing adequate calcium and vitamin D intake for age [7]. According to the Institute of Medicine, in a statement endorsed by the American Academy of Pediatrics and the Society for Adolescent Health and Medicine, for adolescents, the recommended daily intake of calcium is 1300 mg per day and vitamin D is 600 IU per day [76]. In the United States, less than 15 % of adolescent girls meet the daily recommendation for calcium intake and less than one-third for vitamin D intake [77]. Focus on a well-balanced diet with adequate calcium and vitamin D intake should be the goal of physicians when treating their patients who are not meeting the recommended intake of these nutrients [36]. If 25-hydroxyvitamin D level is deficient (<20 ng/mL), it should be corrected by administering 50,000 IU of vitamin D2 or D3 once per week or 2000 IU daily for 6 weeks followed by 400–1000 IU daily to help prevent recurrence [36, 78] . If 25-hydroxyvitamin D level is in the insufficient range (between 20 and 29 ng/dL), evidence is lacking as to whether treatment is needed in healthy adolescents [36], though if needed, the recommended supplementation is 1000 IU per day for at least 3 months [78]. If vitamin D3 is readily available as a supplement, its use is favored by some over vitamin D2 as it may be more potent and have a longer half-life in the body [78].

In general, there is no evidence to broadly recommend pharmacologic treatment for adolescents with the Triad [20]. There are, however, specific situations where medication may be considered although research in this area has primarily focused on adolescents with anorexia nervosa and not on adolescents with the Triad.

If an adolescent athlete has been diagnosed with an eating disorder, psychopharmacologic medications may be considered. There is no evidence to support the use of psychopharmacologic medications in the treatment of adolescents with anorexia nervosa as research has shown that medications are not a useful adjunct to weight restoration and standard intense psychological interventions with respect to weight recovery, weight maintenance, or relapse prevention [79–81]. However, because comorbid psychiatric conditions are common in patients with eating disorders [82, 83], medications may be considered for symptom relief of these comorbid conditions, but it is important to note that symptoms of anxiety and depression in malnourished patients often improve with nutritional rehabilitation [84]. For adolescents with bulimia nervosa, selective serotonin reuptake inhibitors (SSRI) often are used as a successful adjunct to psychotherapy to reduce binge/purge cycle frequency [85].

Combination oral contraceptive (COC) pills have been investigated for their potential role in improving bone health in amenorrheic adolescents through supplementation of exogenous estrogen. Overall, studies of COC in adolescent females with anorexia nervosa have not shown improvement in BMD [86, 87] although a meta-analysis did indicate that COC may attenuate bone loss at the lumbar spine [88]. However due to masking of spontaneous menstrual return, a marker for sufficient energy availability and weight adequacy, as well as lack of extensive evidence for their use, the authors recommended against the use of COCs in these females with anorexia nervosa [88]. Studies in adolescent athletes who are amenorrheic also do not support the use of COC to improve BMD [25, 89]. In all studies, weight gain and menstrual resumption were the factors that were most associated with improved BMD. Because athletes who are amenorrheic have low levels of circulating IGF-1 (a bone trophic hormone) [40], further decreases in IGF-1 levels with COC use likely contributes to this lack of improvement, even with supplemental estrogen.

Transdermal estrogen, because it does not suppress IGF-1 levels, has been investigated as a potential method to increase BMD in adolescents with anorexia nervosa. In a randomized, controlled trial of these patients, transdermal 17β-estradiol at a dose of 100 mcg twice weekly with monthly cyclic progesterone (to prevent unopposed estrogen stimulation of the endometrium) improved BMD at the spine and hip versus the placebo group [90]. To date, transdermal estrogen replacement has not been studied in adolescent athletes; however, the ACSM and Female Athlete Triad coalition recommend consideration of its use in athletes between the ages of 16 and 21 who remain amenorrheic despite at least 1 year of non-pharmacologic therapy, who have low BMD and at least one other Triad risk factor [20].

Another pharmacologic intervention that has been considered in the treatment of adolescent athletes with low BMD is the use of bisphosphonates, which are a class of anti-resorptive agents that inhibit osteoclast function. These medications are most often used in treatment of postmenopausal osteoporosis, but in special circumstances can be used in adolescents. A study of adolescents with anorexia nervosa demonstrated that alendronate may improve BMD in these patients; however, the more important factor in improved BMD was weight restoration [91]. Data are lacking regarding use of bisphosphonates in adolescents with components of the Triad [20]. Because bisphosphonates have a very long half-life and long-term effects in adolescents on both overall health and BMD are largely unknown, these medications should be reserved for very specific conditions such as multiple recurrent fractures, severe pain, or vertebral collapse [36] and not used to treat patients with asymptomatic low BMD [20, 36, 92]. Teriparatide, recombinant parathyroid hormone, an anabolic agent, has been used successfully in a small trial in adult women with anorexia nervosa to improve BMD [93] but has not been studied in adolescents for this purpose.

Recovery

Recovery from the Triad depends largely on the severity of the signs and symptoms when treatment is initiated as more severely affected adolescents typically require a longer duration of time for recovery than those who have more mild manifestations of the Triad. Once energy availability is optimized, recovery of energy status can be as early as days to weeks. Normal menstrual function typically requires months to over a year once energy status has been normalized and recovery of bone health typically requires years [20]. There is some evidence that in adolescents with the Triad, complete recovery of BMD and, ultimately, full realization of genetic peak bone mass accrual do not occur even if energy and menstrual status are restored [7, 49]. For all of these reasons, screening of girls at risk for the Triad is essential.

Screening

To minimize occurrence of adverse consequences of the Triad, early recognition and diagnosis of at risk adolescent athletes is critical [20]. Generally, athletes and coaches are largely unaware of the Triad and its health consequences [94]. A 2011 survey by Feldman et al. demonstrated that over 90 % of surveyed female adolescent athletes did not know of a connection between menstrual function and bone health [95]. Interestingly, coaches routinely observe and note risk factors for the Triad, but often are not knowledgeable about the adverse health consequences and thus may not act on these observations [94]. Because coaches have a unique relationship with their athletes and often their families, they should play a key role in Triad prevention, screening, and education [94].

Currently, in the United States there is no standardized process for screening adolescent girls for components of the Triad. The Female Athlete Triad coalition recommends that screening be part of every pre-participation physical evaluation (PPE) and has recommended a set of 12 questions to use and are as follows [20]:

- Have you ever had a menstrual period?
- How old were you when you had your first menstrual period?
- When was your most recent menstrual period?
- How many periods have you had in the last 12 months?
- Are you presently taking any female hormones (estrogen, progesterone, birth control pills)?
- Do you worry about your weight?
- Are you trying to or has anyone recommended that you gain or lose weight?
- Are you on a special diet or do you avoid certain types of foods or food groups?
- Have you ever had an eating disorder?
- Have you ever had a stress fracture?
- Have you ever been told you have low bone density (osteopenia or osteoporosis)?

Of these questions, 8 of 12 have been incorporated into the 4th edition of the PPE monograph endorsed by multiple organizations including the American Academy of Pediatrics, American Academy of Family Physicians, and the American College of Sports Medicine [96]. This monograph is designed for use with middle school age to collegiate athletes. The efficacy of these 12 questions has not been well studied [97] but the Female Athlete Triad coalition recommends that all female athletes undergo screening with these questions annually [20]. Currently, less than 1/3 of Division I NCAA universities require annual PPE for returning athletes and very few of these universities (less than 10 %) have nine or more of the above questions incorporated into their screening [97]. Screening at the high school level is less clear as less than half of state athletic associations require a single PPE form and far fewer use a form consistent with the 4th edition of the PPE monograph [98]. Other tools for screening female athletes for triad components have been designed [99], but have yet to be widely used.

If an athlete is deemed to be at risk for the Triad based on pre-participation screening, or if a coach, athletic trainer, friend, or family member is concerned about an athlete, prompt referral for evaluation by a qualified medical professional should ensue. With these screening efforts, one of the most important messages is to dispel the myth that amenorrhea or menstrual disturbance is a normal occurrence in female athletes and simply a result of exercise. If parents, coaches, and athletic staff were more aware of this fact, it is likely more adolescents would be brought to attention sooner.

Prevention

As complete recovery of adverse health consequences of the Triad may not be possible, prevention of the Triad becomes an essential part of preventing these consequences. Broad educational initiatives targeting health professionals, coaches, athletic trainers, school administrators, athletes, and families are likely to be the most effective way to prevent the development of the Triad [58]. There have been a limited number of interventional programs designed to prevent Triad components in adolescent athletes with mixed results

[100, 101]. A dissonance-based program that has been successful in eating disorder prevention programs has had positive results in a pilot study that was conducted on the campus of an NCAA-participating school. After participation in this peer-lead program, indicators of eating disorder risk factors were reduced and researchers also found an increase in athletes spontaneously seeking medical evaluation for the Triad [101]. Ongoing study in this area is critical in preventing unintended adverse health consequences in exercising female adolescents.

Outcome

The patient was immediately referred to a sports dietician to assess energy availability and over the course of the next 3 months was able to increase her energy intake gradually and more immediately was able to decrease her exercise to 1 h per day for a month. Once she was able to demonstrate sustained improvement in energy availability, even with exercise, she was allowed to transition to full participation. Ultimately, she was able to increase her BMI to 20.1 (98.5 % of median BMI for age) and at this BMI, 4 months later, she had spontaneous menses. One year later, DXA results showed improved BMD with Z-scores of -1.2 and -1.0 at the spine and total body, respectively.

Clinical Pearls/Pitfalls

1. If an adolescent athlete is identified as having one component of the Triad, evaluation for the other components should follow. Recognition and treatment should not wait until all extremes of the Triad factors are met.
2. Amenorrhea or menstrual irregularity is not normal, even in exercising athletes, and should be evaluated further.
3. Low energy availability can occur in normal weight athletes.

4. A multidisciplinary approach is critical in treating adolescents with the Triad and all members of the team, including the athlete, should have input into the treatment plan.
5. The cornerstone of treatment of the Triad is non-pharmacologic intervention to increase energy availability.
6. Long-term and more immediate adverse health outcomes of the Triad should be discussed; however, an athlete might be more likely to "buy-in" to treatment if the immediate health risks are emphasized.
7. Screening and early diagnosis are key to decreasing long-term health effects of the Triad.

References

1. Garner DM, Olmsted MP, Bohr Y, Garfinkel PE. The eating attitudes test: psychometric features and clinical correlates. Psychol Med. 1982;12:871–8.
2. U.S. Department of Health and Human Services. Physical activity guidelines advisory committee report. Washington, DC: USDHHS; 2008.
3. Zach KN, Smith Machin AL, Hoch AZ. Advances in management of the female athlete triad and eating disorders. Clin Sports Med. 2011;30:551–73.
4. Yeager KK, Agostini R, Nattiv A, Drinkwater B. The female athlete triad: disordered eating, amenorrhea, osteoporosis. Med Sci Sports Exerc. 1993;25:775–7.
5. Nattiv A, Agostini R, Drinkwater B, Yeager KK. The female athlete triad. The inter-relatedness of disordered eating, amenorrhea, and osteoporosis. Clin. Sports Med. 1994;13:405–18.
6. Otis CL, Drinkwater B, Johnson M, Loucks A, Wilmore J. American College of Sports Medicine position stand. The Female Athlete Triad. Med Sci Sports Exerc. 1997;29:i–ix.
7. Nattiv A, Loucks AB, Manore MM, Sanborn CF, Sundgot-Borgen J, Warren MP. American College of Sports Medicine position stand. The female athlete triad. Med Sci Sports Exerc. 2007;39:1867–82.
8. Loucks AB, Kiens B, Wright HH. Energy availability in athletes. J Sports Sci. 2011;29 Suppl 1:S7–15.
9. Loucks AB, Thuma JR. Luteinizing hormone pulsatility is disrupted at a threshold of energy availability in regularly menstruating women. J Clin Endocrinol Metab. 2003;88:297–311.
10. Reed JL, De Souza MJ, Kindler JM, Williams NI. Nutritional practices associated with low energy availability in Division I female soccer players. J Sports Sci. 2014;32:1499–509.

11. Myerson M, Gutin B, Warren MP, May MT, Contento I, Lee M, et al. Resting metabolic rate and energy balance in amenorrheic and eumenorrheic runners. Med Sci Sports Exerc. 1991;23:15–22.
12. De Souza MJ, Lee DK, VanHeest JL, Scheid JL, West SL, Williams NI. Severity of energy-related menstrual disturbances increases in proportion to indices of energy conservation in exercising women. Fertil Steril. 2007;88:971–5.
13. O'Donnell E, Harvey PJ, De Souza MJ. Relationships between vascular resistance and energy deficiency, nutritional status and oxidative stress in oestrogen deficient physically active women. Clin Endocrinol (Oxf). 2009;70:294–302.
14. American Psychiatric Association. Diagnostic and Statistical Manual of Mental Disorders. 5th ed. Arlington, VA: American Psychiatric Publishing; 2013.
15. Gibbs JC, Williams NI, De Souza MJ. Prevalence of individual and combined components of the female athlete triad. Med Sci Sports Exerc. 2013;45:985–96.
16. Holm-Denoma JM, Scaringi V, Gordon KH, Van Orden KA, Joiner TE. Eating disorder symptoms among undergraduate varsity athletes, club athletes, independent exercisers, and nonexercisers. Int J Eat Disord. 2009;42:47–53.
17. Martinsen M, Sundgot-Borgen J. Higher prevalence of eating disorders among adolescent elite athletes than controls. Med Sci Sports Exerc. 2013;45:1188–97.
18. Byrne S, McLean N. Elite athletes: effects of the pressure to be thin. J Sci Med Sport. 2002;5:80–94.
19. Sawaya AL, Tucker K, Tsay R, Willett W, Saltzman E, Dallal GE, et al. Evaluation of four methods for determining energy intake in young and older women: comparison with doubly labeled water measurements of total energy expenditure. Am J Clin Nutr. 1996;63:491–9.
20. Joy E, De Souza MJ, Nattiv A, Misra M, Williams NI, Mallinson RJ, et al. 2014 Female athlete triad coalition consensus statement on treatment and return to play of the female athlete triad. Curr Sports Med Rep. 2014;13:219–32.
21. Rodriguez NR, Di Marco NM, Langley S. American College of Sports Medicine position stand. Nutrition and athletic performance. Med Sci Sports Exerc. 2009;41:709–31.
22. Georgopoulos N, Markou K, Theodoropoulou A, Paraskevopoulou P, Varaki L, Kazantzi Z, et al. Growth and pubertal development in elite female rhythmic gymnasts. J Clin Endocrinol Metab. 1999;84:4525–30.
23. Valentino R, Savastano S, Tommaselli AP, D'Amore G, Dorato M, Lombardi G. The influence of intense ballet training on trabecular bone mass, hormone status, and gonadotropin structure in young women. J Clin Endocrinol Metab. 2001;86:4674–8.
24. Maïmoun L, Coste O, Mura T, Philibert P, Galtier F, Mariano-Goulart D, et al. Specific bone mass acquisition in elite female athletes. J Clin Endocrinol Metab. 2013;98:2844–53.

25. Warren MP, Brooks-Gunn J, Fox RP, Holderness CC, Hyle EP, Hamilton WG, et al. Persistent osteopenia in ballet dancers with amenorrhea and delayed menarche despite hormone therapy: a longitudinal study. Fertil Steril. 2003;80:398–404.
26. Beals KA, Manore MM. Disorders of the female athlete triad among collegiate athletes. Int J Sport Nutr Exerc Metab. 2002;12:281–93.
27. Chumlea WC, Schubert CM, Roche AF, Kulin HE, Lee PA, Himes JH, et al. Age at menarche and racial comparisons in US girls. Pediatrics. 2003;111:110–3.
28. De Souza MJ, Toombs RJ, Scheid JL, O'Donnell E, West SL, Williams NI. High prevalence of subtle and severe menstrual disturbances in exercising women: confirmation using daily hormone measures. Hum Reprod. 2010;25:491–503.
29. Loucks AB, Verdun M, Heath EM. Low energy availability, not stress of exercise, alters LH pulsatility in exercising women. J Appl Physiol. 1998;84:37–46.
30. De Souza MJ, Nattiv A, Joy E, Misra M, Williams NI, Mallinson RJ, et al. 2014 Female Athlete Triad Coalition consensus statement on treatment and return to play of the female athlete triad: 1st International Conference held in San Francisco, CA, May 2012, and 2nd International Conference held in Indianapolis, IN, May 2013. Clin J Sport Med. 2014;24:96–119.
31. Friedman JM, Halaas JL. Leptin and the regulation of body weight in mammals. Nature. 1998;395:763–70.
32. Maïmoun L, Georgopoulos NA, Sultan C. Endocrine disorders in adolescent and young female athletes: impact on growth, menstrual cycles, and bone mass acquisition. J Clin Endocrinol Metab. 2014;99:4037–50.
33. Corr M, De Souza MJ, Toombs RJ, Williams NI. Circulating leptin concentrations do not distinguish menstrual status in exercising women. Hum Reprod. 2011;26:685–94.
34. Osteoporosis prevention, diagnosis, and therapy. NIH Consens Statement. 17:1–45.
35. Bachrach LK. Acquisition of optimal bone mass in childhood and adolescence. Trends Endocrinol Metab. 2001;12:22–8.
36. Golden NH, Abrams SA. Optimizing bone health in children and adolescents. Pediatrics. 2014;134:e1229–43.
37. Hind K, Burrows M. Weight-bearing exercise and bone mineral accrual in children and adolescents: a review of controlled trials. Bone. 2007; 40:14–27.
38. Fehling PC, Alekel L, Clasey J, Rector A, Stillman RJ. A comparison of bone mineral densities among female athletes in impact loading and active loading sports. Bone. 1995;17:205–10.
39. Risser WL, Lee EJ, LeBlanc A, Poindexter HB, Risser JM, Schneider V. Bone density in eumenorrheic female college athletes. Med Sci Sports Exerc. 1990;22:570–4.

40. Christo K, Prabhakaran R, Lamparello B, Cord J, Miller KK, Goldstein MA, et al. Bone metabolism in adolescent athletes with amenorrhea, athletes with eumenorrhea, and control subjects. Pediatrics. 2008;121: 1127–36.
41. Tenforde AS, Fredericson M. Influence of sports participation on bone health in the young athlete: a review of the literature. PM R. 2011;3:861–7.
42. Khosla S, Oursler MJ, Monroe DG. Estrogen and the skeleton. Trends Endocrinol Metab. 2012;23:576–81.
43. Jackowski SA, Erlandson MC, Mirwald RL, Faulkner RA, Bailey DA, Kontulainen SA, et al. Effect of maturational timing on bone mineral content accrual from childhood to adulthood: evidence from 15 years of longitudinal data. Bone. 2011;48:1178–85.
44. Gilsanz V, Chalfant J, Kalkwarf H, Zemel B, Lappe J, Oberfield S, et al. Age at onset of puberty predicts bone mass in young adulthood. J Pediatr. 2011;158:100–5, 105.e1–2.
45. Ihle R, Loucks AB. Dose-response relationships between energy availability and bone turnover in young exercising women. J Bone Miner Res. 2004;19:1231–40.
46. Barrack MT, Rauh MJ, Nichols JF. Cross-sectional evidence of suppressed bone mineral accrual among female adolescent runners. J Bone Miner Res. 2010;25:1850–7.
47. Gibbs JC, Nattiv A, Barrack MT, Williams NI, Rauh MJ, Nichols JF, et al. Low bone density risk is higher in exercising women with multiple triad risk factors. Med Sci Sports Exerc. 2014;46:167–76.
48. Barrack MT, Ackerman KE, Gibbs JC. Update on the female athlete triad. Curr Rev Musculoskelet Med. 2013;6:195–204.
49. Misra M, Prabhakaran R, Miller KK, Goldstein MA, Mickley D, Clauss L, et al. Weight gain and restoration of menses as predictors of bone mineral density change in adolescent girls with anorexia nervosa-1. J Clin Endocrinol Metab. 2008;93:1231–7.
50. Kelsey JL, Bachrach LK, Procter-Gray E, Nieves J, Greendale GA, Sowers M, et al. Risk factors for stress fracture among young female cross-country runners. Med Sci Sports Exerc. 2007;39:1457–63.
51. Bennell KL, Malcolm SA, Thomas SA, Reid SJ, Brukner PD, Ebeling PR, et al. Risk factors for stress fractures in track and field athletes. A twelve-month prospective study. Am J Sports Med. 1996;24:810–8.
52. Korpelainen R, Orava S, Karpakka J, Siira P, Hulkko A. Risk factors for recurrent stress fractures in athletes. Am J Sports Med. 2001;29:304–10.
53. Rauh MJ, Nichols JF, Barrack MT. Relationships among injury and disordered eating, menstrual dysfunction, and low bone mineral density in high school athletes: a prospective study. J Athl Train. 2010;45:243–52.
54. Rauh MJ, Barrack M, Nichols JF. Associations between the female athlete triad and injury among high school runners. Int J Sports Phys Ther. 2014;9:948–58.

55. Nattiv A, Kennedy G, Barrack MT, Abdelkerim A, Goolsby MA, Arends JC, et al. Correlation of MRI grading of bone stress injuries with clinical risk factors and return to play: a 5-year prospective study in collegiate track and field athletes. Am J Sports Med. 2013;41:1930–41.
56. Thijssen DHJ, Black MA, Pyke KE, Padilla J, Atkinson G, Harris RA, et al. Assessment of flow-mediated dilation in humans: a methodological and physiological guideline. Am J Physiol Heart Circ Physiol. 2011; 300:H2–12.
57. O'Donnell E, Goodman JM, Harvey PJ. Clinical review: Cardiovascular consequences of ovarian disruption: a focus on functional hypothalamic amenorrhea in physically active women. J Clin Endocrinol Metab. 2011;96:3638–48.
58. Temme KE, Hoch AZ. Recognition and rehabilitation of the female athlete triad/tetrad: a multidisciplinary approach. Curr Sports Med Rep. 2013;12:190–9.
59. Zeni Hoch A, Dempsey RL, Carrera GF, Wilson CR, Chen EH, Barnabei VM, et al. Is there an association between athletic amenorrhea and endothelial cell dysfunction? Med Sci Sports Exerc. 2003;35:377–83.
60. Rickenlund A, Eriksson MJ, Schenck-Gustafsson K, Hirschberg AL. Amenorrhea in female athletes is associated with endothelial dysfunction and unfavorable lipid profile. J Clin Endocrinol Metab. 2005;90:1354–9.
61. Hoch AZ, Papanek P, Szabo A, Widlansky ME, Schimke JE, Gutterman DD. Association between the female athlete triad and endothelial dysfunction in dancers. Clin J Sport Med. 2011;21:119–25.
62. Herzog DB, Keller MB, Sacks NR, Yeh CJ, Lavori PW. Psychiatric comorbidity in treatment-seeking anorexics and bulimics. J Am Acad Child Adolesc Psychiatry. 1992;31:810–8.
63. Preti A, Rocchi MBL, Sisti D, Camboni MV, Miotto P. A comprehensive meta-analysis of the risk of suicide in eating disorders. Acta Psychiatr Scand. 2011;124:6–17.
64. Keel PK, Dorer DJ, Eddy KT, Franko D, Charatan DL, Herzog DB. Predictors of mortality in eating disorders. Arch Gen Psychiatry. 2003;60:179–83.
65. Steinhausen H-C. Outcome of eating disorders. Child Adolesc Psychiatr Clin N Am. 2009;18:225–42.
66. Arcelus J, Mitchell AJ, Wales J, Nielsen S. Mortality rates in patients with anorexia nervosa and other eating disorders. A meta-analysis of 36 studies. Arch. Gen. Psychiatry. 2011;68:724–31.
67. Gulliver A, Griffiths KM. Mackinnon A. Stanimirovic R. The mental health of Australian elite athletes. J. Sci. Med. Sport: Batterham PJ; 2014.
68. Rosen DS. Identification and management of eating disorders in children and adolescents. Pediatrics. 2010;126:1240–53.
69. Practice Committee of American Society for Reproductive Medicine. Current evaluation of amenorrhea. Fertil Steril. 2008;90:S219–25.

70. House S, Loud K, Shubkin C. Female athlete triad for the primary care pediatrician. Curr Opin Pediatr. 2013;25:755–61.
71. Fairburn CG, Beglin SJ. Assessment of eating disorders: interview or self-report questionnaire? Int J Eat Disord. 1994;16:363–70.
72. Damilakis J, Adams JE, Guglielmi G, Link TM. Radiation exposure in X-ray-based imaging techniques used in osteoporosis. Eur Radiol. 2010;20:2707–14.
73. Lewiecki EM, Gordon CM, Baim S, Leonard MB, Bishop NJ, Bianchi M-L, et al. International Society for Clinical Densitometry 2007 Adult and Pediatric Official Positions. Bone. 2008;43:1115–21.
74. Bishop N, Arundel P, Clark E, Dimitri P, Farr J, Jones G, et al. Fracture prediction and the definition of osteoporosis in children and adolescents: the ISCD 2013 Pediatric Official Positions. J Clin Densitom. 2013;17:275–80.
75. Gordon CM, Bachrach LK, Carpenter TO, Crabtree N, El-Hajj Fuleihan G, Kutilek S, et al. Dual energy X-ray absorptiometry interpretation and reporting in children and adolescents: the 2007 ISCD Pediatric Official Positions. J Clin Densitom. 2007;11:43–58.
76. Institute of Medicine. 2011 Dietary reference intakes for calcium and vitamin D. Washington DC: National Academies Press; 2011.
77. Bailey RL, Dodd KW, Goldman JA, Gahche JJ, Dwyer JT, Moshfegh AJ, et al. Estimation of total usual calcium and vitamin D intakes in the United States. J Nutr. 2010;140:817–22.
78. Society for Adolescent Health and Medicine. Recommended vitamin D intake and management of low vitamin D status in adolescents: a position statement of the society for adolescent health and medicine. J Adolesc Health. 2013;52:801–3.
79. Hagman J, Gralla J, Sigel E, Ellert S, Dodge M, Gardner R, et al. A double-blind, placebo-controlled study of risperidone for the treatment of adolescents and young adults with anorexia nervosa: a pilot study. J Am Acad Child Adolesc Psychiatry. 2011;50:915–24.
80. Holtkamp K, Konrad K, Kaiser N, Ploenes Y, Heussen N, Grzella I, et al. A retrospective study of SSRI treatment in adolescent anorexia nervosa: insufficient evidence for efficacy. J Psychiatr Res. 2005;39:303–10.
81. Kafantaris V, Leigh E, Hertz S, Berest A, Schebendach J, Sterling WM, et al. A placebo-controlled pilot study of adjunctive olanzapine for adolescents with anorexia nervosa. J Child Adolesc Psychopharmacol. 2011;21:207–12.
82. Swanson SA, Crow SJ, Le Grange D, Swendsen J, Merikangas KR. Prevalence and correlates of eating disorders in adolescents. Results from the national comorbidity survey replication adolescent supplement. Arch. Gen. Psychiatry. 2011;68:714–23.
83. Touchette E, Henegar A, Godart NT, Pryor L, Falissard B, Tremblay RE, et al. Subclinical eating disorders and their comorbidity with mood and anxiety disorders in adolescent girls. Psychiatry Res. 2011;185:185–92.

84. Mattar L, Thiébaud M-R, Huas C, Cebula C, Godart N. Depression, anxiety and obsessive-compulsive symptoms in relation to nutritional status and outcome in severe anorexia nervosa. Psychiatry Res. 2012; 200:513–7.

85. Aigner M, Treasure J, Kaye W, Kasper S. World Federation of Societies of Biological Psychiatry (WFSBP) guidelines for the pharmacological treatment of eating disorders. World J Biol Psychiatry. 2011;12:400–43.

86. Golden NH, Lanzkowsky L, Schebendach J, Palestro CJ, Jacobson MS, Shenker IR. The effect of estrogen-progestin treatment on bone mineral density in anorexia nervosa. J Pediatr Adolesc Gynecol. 2002; 15:135–43.

87. Strokosch GR, Friedman AJ, Wu S-C, Kamin M. Effects of an oral contraceptive (norgestimate/ethinyl estradiol) on bone mineral density in adolescent females with anorexia nervosa: a double-blind, placebo-controlled study. J Adolesc Health. 2006;39:819–27.

88. Sim LA, McGovern L, Elamin MB, Swiglo BA, Erwin PJ, Montori VM. Effect on bone health of estrogen preparations in premenopausal women with anorexia nervosa: a systematic review and meta-analyses. Int J Eat Disord. 2010;43:218–25.

89. Cobb KL, Bachrach LK, Sowers M, Nieves J, Greendale GA, Kent KK, et al. The effect of oral contraceptives on bone mass and stress fractures in female runners. Med Sci Sports Exerc. 2007;39:1464–73.

90. Misra M, Katzman D, Miller KK, Mendes N, Snelgrove D, Russell M, et al. Physiologic estrogen replacement increases bone density in adolescent girls with anorexia nervosa. J Bone Miner Res. 2011;26:2430–8.

91. Golden NH, Iglesias EA, Jacobson MS, Carey D, Meyer W, Schebendach J, et al. Alendronate for the treatment of osteopenia in anorexia nervosa: a randomized, double-blind, placebo-controlled trial. J Clin Endocrinol Metab. 2005;90:3179–85.

92. Ducher G, Turner AI, Kukuljan S, Pantano KJ, Carlson JL, Williams NI, et al. Obstacles in the optimization of bone health outcomes in the female athlete triad. Sports Med. 2011;41:587–607.

93. Fazeli PK, Wang IS, Miller KK, Herzog DB, Misra M, Lee H, et al. Teriparatide increases bone formation and bone mineral density in adult women with anorexia nervosa. J Clin Endocrinol Metab. 2014; 99:1322–9.

94. Brown KN, Wengreen HJ, Beals KA. Knowledge of the female athlete Triad, and prevalence of Triad risk factors among female high school athletes and their coaches. J Pediatr Adolesc Gynecol. 2014;27:278–82.

95. Feldmann JM, Belsha JP, Eissa MA, Middleman AB. Female adolescent athletes' awareness of the connection between menstrual status and bone health. J Pediatr Adolesc Gynecol. 2011;24:311–4.

96. American Academy of Pediatrics. In: Bernhardt DT, Roberts WO, editors. Preparticipation physical evaluation. 4th ed. Washington, DC: American Academy of Pediatrics; 2010.

97. Mencias T, Noon M, Hoch AZ. Female athlete triad screening in National Collegiate Athletic Association Division I athletes: is the preparticipation evaluation form effective? Clin J Sport Med. 2012;22:122–5.

98. Madsen NL, Drezner JA, Salerno JC. The preparticipation physical evaluation: an analysis of clinical practice. Clin J Sport Med. 2014;24:142–9.

99. Melin A, Tornberg AB, Skouby S, Faber J, Ritz C, Sjödin A, et al. The LEAF questionnaire: a screening tool for the identification of female athletes at risk for the female athlete triad. Br J Sports Med. 2014;48:540–5.

100. Elliot DL, Goldberg L, Moe EL, Defrancesco CA, Durham MB, McGinnis W, et al. Long-term Outcomes of the ATHENA (Athletes Targeting Healthy Exercise & Nutrition Alternatives) Program for Female High School Athletes. J Alcohol Drug Educ. 2008;52:73–92.

101. Becker CB, McDaniel L, Bull S, Powell M, McIntyre K. Can we reduce eating disorder risk factors in female college athletes? A randomized exploratory investigation of two peer-led interventions. Body Image. 2012;9:31–42.

Chapter 10
Celiac Disease and Abnormal Pubertal Development

Toni Webster and Michael Pettei

Abbreviations

AGA	American Gastroenterological Society
CD	Celiac disease
DHEA-S	Dehydroepiandrosterone sulphate
ELISA	Enzyme-linked immunosorbent assay
EMA-IgA	Anti-endomysial IgA
ESPGHAN	European Society for Pediatric Gastroenterology, Hepatology, and Nutrition
GFD	Gluten-free diet
HLA	Human leukocyte antigen
IEL	Intraepithelial lymphocytes

T. Webster, D.O., M.Sc. (✉) • M. Pettei, M.D., Ph.D.
Division of Pediatric Gastroenterology and Nutrition, Cohen Children's
Medical Center of NY/Long Island Jewish Medical Center,
1991 Marcus Avenue, Lake Success, NY 11042, USA

Hofstra Northwell School of Medicine, Hempstead, NY, USA
e-mail: twebster@nshs.edu; mpettei@nshs.edu

© Springer International Publishing Switzerland 2016 207
H.L. Appelbaum (ed.), *Abnormal Female Puberty*,
DOI 10.1007/978-3-319-27225-2_10

NASPGHAN	North American Society for Pediatric Gastro-enterology, Hepatology, and Nutrition
NIH	National Institutes of Health
TTG-IgA	Tissue transglutaminase IgA

Celia Disease: What Is It?

Introduction

Celiac disease (CD) is a gluten dependent autoimmune enteropathy occurring in those who are genetically susceptible. It has a myriad of clinical presentations. Gastrointestinal symptoms may include abdominal pain, diarrhea, anorexia, weight loss, failure to thrive, vomiting, constipation, and abdominal distention. Extraintestinal manifestations of CD may include dermatitis herpetiformis, dental enamel defects, iron deficiency anemia, aphthous stomatitis, arthritis, arthralgia, short stature, osteoporosis, osteopenia, fractures, and transaminitis. There can also be profound neuropsychiatric symptoms including ataxia, epilepsy, headaches, depression, fatigue, malaise, anxiety, and peripheral neuropathy. However, patients at presentation may lack these findings and only exhibit delayed puberty, irregular menstrual cycles, or prolonged amenorrhea. In older populations, CD may also manifest as infertility or recurrent fetal loss.

Case Presentation

A 16-year-old premenarchal female with no significant past medical history arrives with her mother to a pediatric gastroenterologist for evaluation of poor weight gain and short stature. She has no previous medical history. She has had no surgeries in the past and is not currently taking any prescribed or over-the-counter medications, or herbal supplements. She lives at home with her parents and healthy 13-year-old brother. She excels academically and is involved in many extracurricular activities. She is active, but does not exercise regularly. She denies illicit drug use, alcohol consumption, or sexual activity. Her mother is 5′4″ and her father is 5′11″. Her mother has ulcerative colitis, which is well controlled on mesalamine therapy alone. Multiple members on the maternal side of the family have autoimmune diseases including inflammatory bowel disease, systemic lupus erythematosus, and rheumatoid arthritis. Her father, as well as many of his relatives, has hypercholesterolemia and hypertension.

She maintains a well-rounded diet including dairy products, grains, fruits and vegetables and drinks ample water intake. A typical day will include breakfast, lunch and dinner as well as three snacks. Usually those snacks consist of dietary supplements that are high in calories. She has rare intermittent episodes of abdominal pain. Bowel movements are once to twice daily and soft, but formed, with no visible blood or mucous. She does not have straining or pain with defecation. She admits to excessive flatus and intermittent bloating. She denies steatorrhea, emesis, reflux, weight loss, rashes, mouth ulcers, joint pains, hair loss, and heat or cold intolerance.

On physical examination, her blood pressure and heart rate were within normal limits for age, height 149.5 cm (<3rd%), weight 37.5 kg (<3rd%), and BMI 16.8 kg/m^2 (9th%). She was awake, alert, and in no apparent distress. Her pupils were equally round and reactive to light and her eyes were anicteric. She had a small aphthous ulcer on the right side of her tongue. Her lungs were clear to auscultation and no murmurs were appreciated. Her abdomen was mildly distended, yet, soft and non-tender. No hepatosplenomegaly was appreciated. She was staged as Tanner 5 for breast and pubic hair distribution. Her genital and perianal area appeared normal. On digital rectal examination, there was normal tone and a small amount of soft, guaiac-negative stool in the rectal vault. There were no rashes and the extremities had no clubbing, cyanosis, or edema.

Screening serum laboratory tests included a complete blood cell count, sedimentation rate, c-reactive protein, complete metabolic panel, thyroid stimulating hormone, free thyroxine, tissue transglutaminase IgA, and quantitative immunoglobulin A. They were clinically unremarkable except for a mild microcytic anemia and an elevated tissue transglutaminase IgA > 100 units (nL < 20 units). An upper endoscopy was recommended and revealed the appearance of fissuring of the duodenal mucosa; the stomach and esophagus appeared normal. Histopathology of multiple small bowel biopsies demonstrated the presence of intraepithelial lymphocytosis, moderate villous blunting, and crypt hyperplasia.

Discussion

This patient presented with short stature, poor weight gain, and delayed menarche as well as bloating and frequent flatulence. Her parents are generally of average height and there is a strong history of autoimmune disorders in the family. On physical examination, her weight and height are below the 3rd%, she has an aphthous ulcer of her tongue and her abdomen is mildly distended with gas. If her growth charts were obtained and examined, one would notice that over the past few years she has decreased more than two standard deviations for weight, height, and BMI. Although our patient was likely sent for evaluation of possible inflammatory bowel disease, screening serum laboratory tests did not reveal any elevated inflammatory markers, thrombocytosis, or abnormal albumin level. Instead the recommended screening test for celiac disease, the tissue transglutaminase IgA antibody, was positive with a normal serum IgA level. This test, when strongly positive, indicates the presence of celiac disease but confirmation must be provided by small bowel biopsy. Confirmation of the diagnosis of celiac disease is made evident following demonstration of a response to a gluten-free diet (GFD).

Celiac Disease: How Does It Affect Our Female Population?

While the pathology of CD is defined by the effect on the intestinal tract, multiple systems can be involved. In this case the patient presented with short stature and delayed puberty. The pathogenesis of reproductive dysfunction related to CD is not well understood. Because autoantibodies frequently develop in association with the endocrine glands in CD patients [1–3], some authors have proposed that there may also be antibodies directed against hormones or organs that play a part in pubertal development. After detecting abnormal levels of gonadotropins, others have concluded that the pituitary gland may be a target [4]. Others have hypothesized that abnormal pubertal development in CD may be secondary to increased cytokine production leading to malabsorption of essential nutrients that are integral in signaling and transport of sex hormones [5]. Significantly lower levels of dehydroepiandrosterone sulphate (DHEA-S) were reported in untreated CD patients compared to their counterparts adhering to a gluten-free diet (GFD). Furthermore, both CD groups had significantly lower levels of DHEA-S with respect to controls [6]. DHEA has been shown to inhibit proinflammatory cytokines such as secretion of tumor necrosis factor [7–11] and interleukin 6 [12–14].

Menarche may occur significantly later in untreated girls with CD compared to girls without CD or girls on a strict GFD [15, 16]. After menarche occurs, up to 60 % will suffer from an irregular menstrual cycle. In one study, after six to eight months of treatment with a GFD, cycles normalized in girls with CD [16].

Clinical and epidemiological studies have demonstrated the negative effects of untreated CD on pregnancy including higher risks of fetal intrauterine growth retardation, shorter duration of pregnancy, low birth weight, and reduced duration of lactation. Not only are pregnancies three times more likely to be spontaneously aborted in females with untreated CD [16], individuals with CD are at an increased risk for repeated spontaneous abortions [17]. This has led some researchers to conclude that asymptomatic celiac disease should be suspected and screened in otherwise healthy females with multiple abortions [18]. Females with untreated CD, who previously had repeated spontaneous abortions, were able to conceive and give birth to healthy full-term infants when strictly adhering to a GFD [16].

Females with untreated CD and pubertal delay will consequently also have a shorter period of fertility. This is further compounded by the observation that untreated females with CD have a tendency to suffer from premature ovarian insufficiency in comparison to girls without CD. However, it was shown that fertile life span was extended if a GFD was started at least 10 years prior to menopause. Aside from an association with early menopause, untreated CD is linked to an increased risk of menopause-associated disorders. Women who are untreated are more likely to experience hot flashes, muscle aches, joint problems, and irritability. Symptoms of muscle aches and joint problems significantly improve with institution of a GFD [19].

The effect of CD on puberty as it relates to growth, failure to thrive, and short stature has been well described and evidenced. Short stature is often one of the presenting symptoms of CD; those with isolated stunted growth or short stature have been calculated to have a 10–40 % risk of CD [20, 21]. Institution of a GFD generally results in normalization of nutritional measures, growth acceleration, and improvement in weight. The effect of a GFD on protein, fat, and bone compartments in children with CD was studied by assessing height, arm muscle area, triceps skinfolds, subscapular skinfolds, fat area index, and bone mineral content before and after adherence to a GFD. After 1 year on a GFD, the only statistical differences found between children on a GFD and healthy controls were height and arm muscle area [22, 23]. Another study that evaluated body composition in children with CD on a GFD reexamined them after 4 years. Height, bone mineral content, fat mass, and bone mineral density normalized, yet weight and fat-free mass remained lower [24]. Interestingly, it was shown that the final adult height of female patients with CD is similar to the general population regardless of whether diagnosis occurred prior to or after 18 years of age. The same could not be said for their male counterparts in the study, whose adult height was inversely related to age of diagnosis [25].

Epidemiology and Genetics

In Europe and North America, the current prevalence of CD is approximately 1 % [26, 27] with the highest prevalence worldwide in Saharawi children [28]. Females are more commonly affected, with approximately twice the likelihood to have CD in comparison to their male counterparts. A genetic susceptibility to CD is demonstrated by an approximately 10 % risk for CD in first degree relatives of those diagnosed [29]. While genetic factors play an important role, they are not the only factor in CD development. In fact, there is only 75 % concordance rate in monozygotic twins [30]. The strongest genetic susceptibility to CD maps to the human leukocyte antigen (HLA) region on chromosome 6, including class II genes HLA-DQ2 and HLA-DQ8. An individual with CD may possess either the HLA-DQ2 or DQ8 genes (or a portion of the haplotype). HLA class II genes, also referred to as CELIAC1, explain only a portion of disease heritability. Other non-HLA genetic risk factor regions have been described in genetic linkage analysis studies including CELIAC2 on 5q31–33 [31], CELIAC3 on 2q33 [32], and CELIAC4 on 19p13.1 [33]. Genome-wide association studies have identified multiple loci associated with CD, many of these are also implicated in type 1 diabetes [34]. These non-HLA loci are considered to impart a comparatively small portion of overall genetic risk.

There is an increased incidence of CD in patients with type 1 diabetes, autoimmune thyroiditis, autoimmune liver disease, IgA deficiency, Down syndrome, Turner syndrome, Williams syndrome and those with a first degree relative with CD. Thus it is recommended by the North American Society for Pediatric Gastroenterology, Hepatology, and Nutrition (NASPGHAN) to screen patients who are considered to be at increased risk starting at 3 years of age as long as they have been ingesting an adequate gluten load for at least 1 year prior to testing [35]. Screening can be repeated later in life regardless of a prior negative screening result because CD may develop over time. Less frequently, there is an association noted between CD and Addison's disease, Sjogren's syndrome, pernicious anemia, autoimmune thrombocytopenia, sarcoidosis, alopecia areata, vitiligo, psoriasis, hepatitis, cholangitis, and autoimmune cardiomyopathy. These comorbidities alone are not considered reasons for screening unless otherwise clinically indicated.

Diagnosis: From Blood to Biopsies

Diagnostic criteria vary between professional societies of gastroenterologists including NASPGHAN, the European Society for Pediatric Gastroenterology, Hepatology, and Nutrition (ESPGHAN), the National Institutes of Health (NIH) and the American

Gastroenterological Society (AGA). However, they do agree that
serologic testing is the first step when evaluating a symptomatic
patient. Tissue transglutaminase IgA (TTG-IgA) is performed by an
enzyme-linked immunosorbent assay (ELISA) and is recommended
as the initial serologic test for CD [35, 36] given its high sensitivity
and specificity [37]. An immunofluorescent technique is implemented in the measurement of anti-endomysial IgA (EMA-IgA)
and is theoretically as accurate as TTG-IgA; however, the operator
dependent interpretation of the immunofluorescence may lead to
inaccuracy and performance of the EMA-IgA is more costly. Antigliadin antibodies are no longer a recommended diagnostic test for
CD given the low specificity and high false negative rate; although,
there is evidence to suggest the usefulness of this assay in children
younger than 2 years of age [38]. The newer deamidated gliadin
peptide antibody assay outperforms its predecessor; however, in
comparison TTG-IgA and EMA-IgA are still superior. The important celiac antibodies include all IgA antibodies and a quantitative
immunoglobulin A level to confirm accuracy. It is important to consider that IgA deficiency is a condition associated 10 % of the time
with celiac disease. For those with serum IgA deficiency, the less
sensitive and specific IgG antibodies must be assessed. A false-
negative TTG-IgA may occur even with a normal IgA as a result of
ingestion of a low gluten containing diet, concomitant protein losing enteropathy, immunosuppressive therapy, or if the patient is
younger than 2 years of age [36].

Once positive serologic testing is identified, biopsies attained
via upper endoscopy or suction capsule are necessary to confirm
diagnosis by histopathology according to NASPGHAN guidelines
[35]. The ESPGHAN guidelines differ slightly in that a biopsy
proven diagnosis may not be required in specific pediatric patients
with typical overt signs or symptoms of CD. If a TTG-IgA level is
greater than 10 times the upper limit of normal, and EMA and HLA
testing are performed and compatible with celiac disease, a GFD
can be instituted [36]. Close observation demonstrating resolution
of symptoms and celiac antibodies could then confirm the diagnosis. This method of diagnosis would not be applicable to asymptomatic children or those with atypical symptoms who are not able
to demonstrate a clear-cut clinical response. Antibody negative

celiac disease can occur even in the face of normal IgA levels. Thus, individuals with symptoms compatible with CD and negative serologic tests should be considered for further diagnostic investigation including intestinal biopsy.

When CD diagnosis is uncertain, obtaining HLA class II genes HLA-DQ2 and HLA-DQ8 may be considered. A positive test is not useful since it is present in 30–40 % of the general population, but 99 % of individuals with celiac disease possess a DQ2 or DQ8 marker. Because of a high negative predictive value, a negative HLA test virtually excludes the diagnosis of CD.

When tissue diagnosis is required, multiple small bowel biopsies are taken from the duodenal bulb and distal duodenum to increase the likelihood of attaining characteristic histology given the patchy nature of CD. Classic histology of CD consists of variable amounts of villous blunting, with the most severe being "flat" mucosa, combined with crypt hyperplasia and increased intraepithelial lymphocytes (Fig. 10.1). A grading system has been developed to provide pathologists with a consistent method of reporting histologic findings [39]; however, it is important to recognize that these findings are not pathognomonic for CD. The clinical setting is important since these biopsy changes may also be seen with milk-protein allergy, intractable diarrhea of infancy, infection, primary immunodeficiencies, and intestinal lymphoma. Diagnosis of CD requires a response to the institution of a GFD in a patient with characteristic changes on small bowel biopsy. A response may consist of resolution of symptoms or, for the asymptomatic individual,

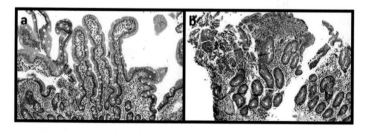

Fig. 10.1 Histologic features of CD, hematoxylin and eosin stain. (**a**) Normal duodenal biopsy with tall slender villi and normal number of intraepithelial lymphocytes, 100× magnification. (**b**) Duodenal biopsy demonstrating villous blunting and increased number of intraepithelial lymphocytes, 100× magnification

the resolution of the celiac antibodies. In difficult cases, small bowel biopsy should be repeated to document changes.

Management: Present and Future

The mainstay of treatment for celiac disease is the complete elimination of all gluten from the diet. Gluten and related proteins are present in wheat, barley, and rye (Fig. 10.2) [40]. Triticale, kamut, and spelt should be avoided as well as malt which is derived from barley. Although oats themselves are naturally gluten free, one must be cautious since cross contamination can occur when oats are milled in a location that also produces wheat, barley, or rye. In addition to overt grain products, gluten is often added to many products and thus appears in items not generally associated with grain products or even as food. One must pay particular attention to the labeling on packaged products. A registered dietitian experienced in providing education and guidance for patients with CD is essential in the initial counseling.

On August 5th, 2014, the final rule on gluten-free labeling that was originally published in August 2013 by the US Food and Drug Administration took effect. The final rule provides a uniform standard definition as to what foods may be labeled "gluten-free," which includes if they are inherently gluten free or they contain less than 20 ppm of gluten [41]. Cross contamination may not only happen during processing and transportation of food prior to its arrival in the home, but unintentionally during meal preparation within the home as well. Special care must be taken in placing gluten-free and gluten-containing items in separate pantries, and using two sets of items such as toasters which cannot be practically cleaned of gluten products. Other culprits that may harbor gluten are toothpaste and over the counter as well as prescribed medications, including vitamins. Some cosmetic products applied to the lips, including lip balm, gloss, and lipstick, contain trace amounts of gluten. There is currently no evidence of transdermal absorption of gluten, so other cosmetics, lotions, oils and creams as well as artistic mediums are not suspect.

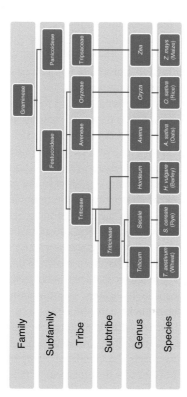

Fig. 10.2 Taxonomic relationships of major cereal grains. Adapted from Kasarda DD [34]

When initiating a GFD in a patient with more severe disease, a temporary lactose free diet may improve symptoms since transient lactase deficiency is associated with villous atrophy. During the initial diagnosis of celiac disease consideration needs to be given to screening for anemia and, when appropriate, various vitamin levels. Supplementation with a GF vitamin supplement is recommended not only to ameliorate potential inadequacies at presentation but to partially replace the B-vitamin supplementation that is provided in wheat products. At diagnosis of CD, one may consider assessing Hepatitis B antibody status since patients with CD are associated with a lower rate of appropriate immune response to the primary Hepatitis B virus vaccine series [42].

While presently the only effective treatment for celiac disease is the initiation of a life-long GFD, there are many potential treatments on the horizon that may either substitute for the diet or provide temporary respite from diet. Various polypeptide sequences derived from gluten proteins are able to reach the lamina propria since they are resistant to enzymatic digestion in the gastrointestinal tract, a factor that likely contributes to the immunogenicity of gluten peptides. Therefore, one of the areas of investigation in CD treatment relates to proteases that will degrade and thus ultimately detoxify gluten, appropriately termed glutenases. ALV003, a mixture of highly specific glutenases, has been shown to block immune responses induced by gluten in patients with celiac disease. However, symptoms caused by gluten consumption were still reported even with pretreatment with ALV003 [43]. *Aspergillus niger* prolyl endoprotease (AN-PEP), a glutenase that is a post-proline cutting enzyme, allowed only a minimal amount of gluten-derived polypeptides to reach the duodenal compartment in a gastrointestinal model [44]. Future development of these proteases may ultimately comprise adjunctive therapy and allow intermittent gluten consumption for patients with CD. A polymeric binder that neutralizes immunogenicity by forming a complex with gluten in a mouse model has also been investigated [45, 46].

HLA blockers are another area of interest in CD treatment. HLA DQ2 and DQ8 molecules present modified gluten peptides to T-cells yielding activated helper cells. If these sites are blocked, gluten is never presented and T-cell activation cannot occur. Blocking the gluten peptide-binding site of HLA-DQ2 with two types of peptide analogues modeled after gluten has been studied. T cell receptor recognition of peptide-DQ2 was inhibited and one peptide analogue was found to be effective at inhibiting antigen presentation [47].

Zonulin has been shown to increase trans-epithelial permeability and to be increased in the intestinal tissue of patients with CD compared to healthy controls. Larazotide acetate, a zonulin antagonist that prevents tight junction opening, reduced gluten-immune reactivity and symptoms in CD patients undergoing gluten challenge. Measures of intestinal permeability did not differ between those using larazotide acetate and the placebo group [46, 48].

TTG plays a critical role in celiac disease pathogenesis by unmasking normally hidden epitopes via deamidation. It is hypothesized that TTG inhibitors may be well tolerated in humans given that TTG-null mice seem to be unaffected. Multiple small molecule TTG inhibitors have been studied [49, 50].

The concept of protein desensitization often used in the field of allergy is being applied with peptide constituents as immunotherapy to induce gluten tolerance in CD. Nexvax2, a prototypical synthetic gluten peptide vaccine, is based on HLA-DQ2 recognition and is currently undergoing clinical trials. If peptide desensitization is a success, another vaccine will require design for those patients with HLA-DQ8 since T-cell epitopes differ based on HLA gene class [46, 51].

Decreasing inflammatory cytokines is another potential therapeutic strategy in CD. Current investigations include anti-interferon gamma antibody and antibody-mediated blockade of IL-15. Other targets in the immune pathogenesis cascade being studied are anti-CD3 and anti-CD20 monoclonal antibodies as well as chemokine receptor CCR9 antagonists [52].

There have been strides in developing a dietary therapy by breeding barley and wheat varieties that lack gluten. There are already some strains that naturally exist that lack some but not all of the immunogenic peptides. A genetically modified variety was engineered with transcriptional suppression of the major source of immunogenic epitopes using RNA interference. There was significant reduction in the amount of immunogenic prolamins in this wheat strain [46, 53]. How modification affects feasibility of mass production, cost, and palatability is unknown at this time.

Outcomes

The family received dietary education, which was provided by a nutritionist, and the patient initiated a strict GFD. Over the next few months the patient experienced complete resolution of symptoms followed by rapid weight gain and increase in growth velocity and menarche was achieved. By her 17th birthday her menstrual cycle had completely normalized and by her 18th birthday her height was 155 cm (5th%), weight was 47 kg (9th%), and BMI was 21.3 kg/m^2 (33rd%).

Clinical Pearls and Pitfalls

1. CD should be considered in females with abnormal puberty and reproductive dysfunction.
2. The recommended screening test for CD is TTG-IgA in an individual with a normal serum IgA level.
3. CD is confirmed by small bowel biopsy; however, a response to GFD diet must be demonstrated for diagnosis of CD.
4. Although there are many potential treatments for CD, a GFD is the mainstay of treatment.
5. Final adult height of female patients with CD on a GFD is similar to the general population regardless of time to diagnosis or initiation of GFD.
6. Menarche occurs later in females with untreated CD versus those on a strict GFD or those without CD.
7. Menstrual cycles in females with CD normalized after 6–8 months of a GFD.

References

1. Di Mario U, Anastasi E, Mariani P, et al. Diabetes-related autoantibodies do appear in children with coeliac disease. Acta Paediatr. 1992;81:593–7.
2. Scott BB, Losowski MS. Coeliac disease: a cause of various associated disease? Lancet. 1975;ii:956–7.

3. Velluzzi F, Caradonna A, Boy MF, et al. Thyroid and celiac disease: clinical, serological and echographic study. Am J Gastroenterol. 1998;93:976–9.

4. Collin P, Hakanen M, Salmi J, Mäki M, Kaukinen K. Autoimmune hypopituitarism in patients with coeliac disease: symptoms confusingly similar. Scand J Gastroenterol. 2001;36:558–60.

5. Bona G, Marinello D, Oderda G. Mechanisms of abnormal puberty in coeliac disease. Horm Res. 2002;57 Suppl 2:63–5.

6. Toscano V, Conti FG, Anastasi E, et al. Importance of gluten in the induction of endocrine autoantibodies and organ dysfunction in adolescent celiac patients. Am J Gastroenterol. 2000;95(7):1742–8.

7. Danenberg HD, Alpert G, Lustig S, et al. Dehydroepiandrosterone protects mice from endotoxin toxicity and reduces tumor necrosis factor production. Antimicrob Agents Chemother. 1992;36(10):2275–9.

8. Di Santo E, Foddi MC, Ricciardi-Castagnoli P, et al. DHEAS inhibits TNF production in monocytes, astrocytes and microglial cells. Neuroimmunomodulation. 1996;3(5):285–8.

9. Araghi-Niknam M, Zhang Z, Jiang S, et al. Cytokine dysregulation and increased oxidation is prevented by dehydroepiandrosterone in mice infected with murine leukemia retrovirus. Proc Soc Exp Biol Med. 1997;216(3):386–91.

10. Kimura M, Tanaka S, Yamada Y, et al. Dehydroepiandrosterone decreases serum tumor necrosis factor-alpha and restores insulin sensitivity: independent effect from secondary weight reduction in genetically obese Zucker fatty rats. Endocrinology. 1998;139(7):3249–53.

11. Padgett DA, Loria RM. Endocrine regulation of murine macrophage function: effects of dehydroepiandrosterone, androstenediol, and androstenetriol. J Neuroimmunol. 1998;84(1):61–8.

12. Daynes RA, Araneo BA, Ershler WB, et al. Altered regulation of IL-6 production with normal aging. Possible linkage to the age-associated decline in dehydroepiandrosterone and its sulfated derivative. J Immunol. 1993;150(12):5219–30.

13. Straub RH, Konecna L, Hrach S, et al. Serum dehydroepiandrosterone (DHEA) and DHEA sulfate are negatively correlated with serum interleukin-6 (IL-6), and DHEA inhibits IL-6 secretion from mononuclear cells in man in vitro: possible link between endocrinosenescence and immunosenescence. J Clin Endocrinol Metab. 1998;83(6):2012–7.

14. Gordon CM, LeBoff MS, Glowacki J. Adrenal and gonadal steroids inhibit IL-6 secretion by human marrow cells. Cytokine. 2001;16(5):178–86.

15. Rujner J. Age at menarche in girls with celiac disease. Ginekol Pol. 1999;70(5):359–62.

16. Bykova SV, Sabel'nikova EA, Parfenov AI, et al. Reproductive disorders in women with celiac disease. Effect of the etiotropic therapy. Eksp Klin Gastroenterol. 2011;3:12–8.

17. Molteni N, Bardella MT, Bianchi PA. Obstetric and gynecological problems in women with untreated celiac sprue. J Clin Gastroenterol. 1990; 12(1):37–9.

18. Foschi F, Diani F, Zardini E, et al. Celiac disease and spontaneous abortion. Minerva Ginecol. 2002;54(2):151–9.
19. Santonicola A, Iovino P, Cappello C, et al. From menarche to menopause: the fertile life span of celiac women. Menopause. 2011;18(10):1125–30.
20. Bottaro G, Cataldo F, Rotolo N, et al. The clinical pattern of subclinical/silent celiac disease: an analysis on 1026 consecutive cases. Am J Gastroenterol. 1999;94:691–6.
21. van Rijn JC, Grote FK, Oostdijk W, et al. Short stature and the probability of coeliac disease, in the absence of gastrointestinal symptoms. Arch Dis Child. 2004;89:882–3.
22. Calaco J, Egan-Mitchell B, Stevens FM, et al. Compliance with gluten free diet in coeliac disease. Arch Dis Child. 1987;62:706–8.
23. Rea F, Polito C, Marotta A, et al. Restoration of body composition in celiac children after one year of gluten-free diet. J Pediatr Gastroenterol Nutr. 1996;23:408–12.
24. Carbone MC, Pitzalis G, Ferri M, et al. Body composition in coeliac disease adolescents on a gluten-free diet: a longitudinal study. Acta Diabetol. 2003;40 Suppl 1:S171–3.
25. Weiss B, Skourikhin Y, Modan-Moses D, et al. Is adult height of patients with celiac disease influenced by delayed diagnosis? Am J Gastroenterol. 2008;103(7):1770–4.
26. Fasano A, Berti I, Gerarduzzi T, et al. Prevalence of celiac disease in at-risk and not-at-risk groups in the United States: a large multicenter study. Arch Intern Med. 2003;163(3):286–92.
27. Mustalahti K, Catassi C, Reunanen A, et al. The prevalence of celiac disease in Europe: results of a centralized, international mass screening project. Ann Med. 2010;42(8):587–95.
28. Catassi C, Rätsch IM, Gandolfi L, et al. Why is coeliac disease endemic in the people of the Sahara? Lancet. 1999;354(9179):647–8.
29. Mäki M, Holm K, Lipsanen V, et al. Serological markers and HLA genes among healthy first-degree relatives of patients with coeliac disease. Lancet. 1991;338:1350–3.
30. Nisticò L, Fagnani C, Coto I, et al. Concordance, disease progression, and heritability of coeliac disease in Italian twins. Gut. 2006;55(6):803–8.
31. Greco L, Corazza G, Babron MC, et al. Genome search in celiac disease. Am J Hum Genet. 1998;62(3):669–75.
32. Djilali-Saiah I, Schmitz J, Harfouch-Hammoud E, et al. CTLA-4 gene polymorphism is associated with predisposition to celiac disease. Gut. 1998;43(2):187–9.
33. BelzenVan MJ, Meijer JW, Sandkuijl LA, et al. A major non-HLA locus in celiac disease maps to chromosome 19. Gastroenterology. 2003;125(4): 1032–41.
34. Smyth DJ, Plagnol V, Walker NM, et al. Shared and distinct genetic variants in Type 1 diabetes and celiac disease. N Engl J Med. 2008;359(26):2767–77.

35. Hill ID, Dirks MH, Liptak GS, et al. Guideline for the diagnosis and treatment of celiac disease in children: recommendations of the North American Society for Pediatric Gastroenterology, Hepatology and Nutrition. J Pediatr Gastroenterol Nutr. 2005;40(1):1–19.

36. Husby S, Koletzko S, Korponay-Szabó IR, et al. European Society for Pediatric Gastroenterology, Hepatology, and Nutrition guidelines for the diagnosis of coeliac disease. J Pediatr Gastroenterol Nutr. 2012;54(1):136–60.

37. Sulkanen S, Halttunen T, Laurila K, et al. Tissue transglutaminase autoantibody enzyme-linked immunosorbent assay in detecting celiac disease. Gastroenterology. 1998;115(6):1322–8.

38. Lagerqvist C, Dahlbom I, Hansson T, et al. Antigliadin immunoglobulin A best in finding celiac disease in children younger than 18 months of age. J Pediatr Gastroenterol Nutr. 2008;47(4):428–35.

39. Oberhuber G, Granditsch G, Vogelsang H. The histopathology of coeliac disease: time for a standardized report scheme for pathologists. Eur J Gastroenterol Hepatol. 1999;11(10):1185–94.

40. Kasarda DD. Gluten and gliadin: precipitating factors in coeliac disease. In: Mäki M, Collin P, Visakorpi JK, editors. Coeliac disease. Proceedings of the seventh international symposium on coeliac disease. Tampere: Coeliac Disease Study Group, University of Tampere; 1997. p. 195–212.

41. U.S. Food and Drug Administration [Internet]. Silver Spring: U.S. Food and Drug Administration; 2014 [updated 2014 August 5, cited 2015 February 14]. http://www.fda.gov/Food/NewsEvents/ConstituentUpdates/ucm407867.htm

42. Park SD, Markowitz J, Pettei M, et al. Failure to respond to hepatitis B vaccine in children with celiac disease. J Pediatr Gastroenterol Nutr. 2007;44(4):431–5.

43. Tye-Din JA, Anderson RP, Ffrench RA, et al. The effects of ALV003 pre-digestion of gluten on immune response and symptoms in celiac disease in vivo. Clin Immunol. 2010;134(3):289–95.

44. Mitea C, Havenaar R, Drijfhout JW, et al. Efficient degradation of gluten by a prolyl endoprotease in a gastrointestinal model: implications for coeliac disease. Gut. 2008;57(1):25–32.

45. Pinier M, Verdu EF, Nasser-Eddine M, et al. Polymeric binders suppress gliadin-induced toxicity in the intestinal epithelium. Gastroenterology. 2009;136(1):288–98.

46. Fasano A. Clinical guide to gluten-related disorders. 1st ed. Philadelphia: Lippincott Williams & Wilkins; 2013.

47. Xia J, Bergseng E, Fleckenstein B, et al. Cyclic and dimeric gluten peptide analogues inhibiting DQ2 mediated antigen presentation in coeliac disease. Bioorg Med Chem. 2007;15(20):6565–73.

48. Kelly CP, Green PH, Murray JA, et al. Larazotide acetate in patients with coeliac disease undergoing a gluten challenge: a randomized placebo-controlled study. Aliment Pharmacol Ther. 2013;37(2):252–62.

49. Watts RE, Siegel M, Khosla C. Structure-activity relationship analysis of the selective inhibition of transglutaminase 2 by dihydroisoxazoles. J Med Chem. 2006;49:7493–501.
50. Duval E, Case A, Stein RL, Cuny GD. Structure-activity relationship study of novel tissue transglutaminase inhibitors. Bioorg Med Chem Lett. 2005;15:1885–9.
51. Tye-Din JA, Stewart JA, Dromey JA, et al. Comprehensive, quantitative mapping of T cell epitopes in gluten in coeliac disease. Sci Transl Med. 2010;2:41ra51.
52. Sollid LM, Khosla CJ. Novel therapies for coeliac disease. Intern Med. 2011;269(6):604–13.
53. Wen S, Wen N, Pang J, et al. Structural genes of wheat and barley 5-methylcytosine DNA glycosylases and their potential applications for human health. Proc Natl Acad Sci U S A. 2012;109(50):20543–8.

Chapter 11
Ovarian Neoplasms and Abnormal Pubertal Development

Jill S. Whyte

Case

A 16-year-old girl presented to her pediatrician with a complaint of abdominal pain. She reports that the pain started approximately 1 month ago and has gradually worsened in severity. The patient's mother notes the development of acne and coarse hair on the patient's abdomen and upper lip.

Past medical history is unremarkable. All developmental milestones have been achieved normally patient's. The patient had not started menstruating, although breast development began at age 11 years. She denies a history of sexual activity.

Examination demonstrates a thin, anxious appearing adolescent. Breast and pubic hair development was Tanner stage 5. Sparse dark hairs were noted on the face and abdomen. The abdomen was noted to be distended with a palpable mass in the lower abdomen.

J.S. Whyte, M.D. (✉)
Division of Gynecologic Oncology, North Shore University Hospital, 10 Monti, 300 Community Drive, Manhasset, NY, 11030, USA

Hofstra Northwell School of Medicine, Hempstead, NY, USA
e-mail: jwhyte@nshs.edu

© Springer International Publishing Switzerland 2016
H.L. Appelbaum (ed.), *Abnormal Female Puberty*,
DOI 10.1007/978-3-319-27225-2_11

The patient underwent abdominal ultrasound which revealed a 16 cm cystic and solid mass arising from the left adnexa. A normal appearing right ovary and uterus were identified. She underwent contrast enhanced CT scans of the abdomen and pelvis which confirmed the presence of an enhancing complex cystic and solid pelvic mass and scant ascites.

Discussion

This is a 16-year-old female who presents with amenorrhea, signs of virilization, and a large, complex pelvic mass suggestive of malignancy. Ovarian tumors are uncommon in children with an incidence of 2.6 cases per 100,000 girls per year [1]. The differential diagnosis is broad and includes benign and malignant ovarian neoplasms. Malignancy is reported in 10–15 % of ovarian masses and comprises 1–2 % of childhood malignancies [2]. Physiologic ovarian cysts are uncommon in prepubertal children but become more common in adolescents. Most simple ovarian cysts, however, are physiologic, result from follicular enlargement, and will resolve spontaneously.

Ovarian tumors that occur in childhood and adolescence include ovarian germ cell tumors (OGCT), sex cord stromal tumors (SCST), small cell carcinomas, epithelial tumors and leukemia and lymphoma. The distribution of tumor types is clearly different in the pediatric compared to adult population. Germ cell tumors are the most common type of pediatric ovarian tumor, followed by stromal and epithelial neoplasms [3]. Precocious puberty occurs in fewer than 10 % of patients presenting with a childhood ovarian malignancy [4]. Patients commonly present with abdominal pain and a palpable abdominal mass [5]. Other presenting symptoms can include nausea and vomiting, constipation, urinary frequency, or signs of virilization.

In young girls with a suspected ovarian mass, transabdominal ultrasound is the imaging modality of choice. Transvaginal sonography may be performed in sexually active adolescents. Sonography can determine whether a mass is cystic or solid, simple or complex, unilateral or bilateral. The presence of ascites or abnormal ovarian blood flow on Doppler studies may raise the index of suspicion for malignancy. Large mass size (>10 cm), solid components, and elevated tumor markers are predictive of malignancy [6]. Assessment of serum tumor markers may help to narrow the differential diagnosis; however, tumor markers are positive in only 50 % of patients presenting with malignancy [7]. Serum alpha-fetoprotein (AFP) is elevated in patients with endodermal sinus tumors, embryonal carcinomas, and immature teratomas. Lactate dehydrogenase (LDH) is elevated in dysgerminomas. Human chorionic gonadotropin (HCG) is elevated in choriocarcinoma and embryonal carcinomas. Inhibin is elevated in granulosa cell tumors and some Sertoli–Leydig cell tumors. Estrogen and testosterone may be secreted by ovarian stromal tumors resulting in menstrual irregularities or delayed menarche. CA 125 is a sensitive marker for the presence of ovarian epithelial cancer; however, CA 125 lacks specificity and may be elevated in a variety of benign gynecologic and non-gynecologic conditions.

Acute onset of abdominal pain should in the presence of an abdominal or pelvic mass should raise suspicion for ovarian torsion. Torsion may be more common in benign rather than malignant ovarian neoplasms, particularly in children and adolescents [8]. In one study of 102 girls (aged 9.8 ± 5.5 years; range, 2 days to 20 years) undergoing ovarian surgery, 42 % (25/59) of patients presenting with acute abdominal pain had an ovarian torsion and one had a malignant ovarian neoplasm in contrast to those presenting with an asymptomatic mass of whom 26 % (6/23) had malignancies [9]. Ultrasound is the imaging modality of choice in young women suspected of ovarian torsion. The reported sensitivity of ultrasound for the diagnosis of torsion ranges from 46 to 75 % [10, 11]. Surgery should not be delayed in children and adolescents suspected of ovarian torsion, regardless of the ultrasound findings, as the ovary can often be salvaged. A laparoscopic approach is feasible in most cases.

Germ Cell Tumors of the Ovary

Germ cell tumors are the most common ovarian neoplasms in children and young women [12] and may be benign or malignant. Benign mature cystic teratomas are the most common OGCT. Mature cystic teratomas characteristically appear on ultrasound as a cystic mass containing fat. A densely echogenic peripheral nodule may be seen (Rokitansky nodule) and frequently contains calcifications [13]. Treatment in children and adolescents consists of fertility preserving excision, preferably with laparoscopy and ovarian cystectomy. Autoimmune paraneoplastic syndromes such as anti-NMDA receptor limbic encephalitis have been reported with benign teratomas [14]. Malignant degeneration of dermoid components into a somatic malignant neoplasm occurs in fewer than 2 % of mature cystic teratomas and is more common in the adult population [15].

OGCT are derived from the primordial germ cells of the ovary and comprise approximately 20–25 % of all ovarian neoplasms. Only 3 % of germ cell tumors are malignant, and malignant ovarian germ cell tumors (MOGCT) account for less than 5 % of all ovarian malignancies. These tumors arise primarily in young women in the second and third decade of life with a peak incidence between ages 16 and 20 [16]. MOGCT are rare in premenarchal girls, accounting for fewer than 20 % of MOGCT and less than 1 % of malignant childhood tumors [17]. Germ cell malignancies may grow rapidly and are often associated with hormonal or enzymatic activity. Patients may present with precocious puberty, but more commonly present with pain, abdominal distention, or symptoms that mimick pregnancy.

Dysgerminoma is the most common malignant germ cell tumor in children and young women, followed by immature teratoma, endodermal sinus tumor, and mixed germ cell tumors [15]. Pelvic imaging typically demonstrates a large predominantly solid or mixed cystic and solid mass in the pelvis. Dysgerminoma classically appears as a multilobulated, solid, large adnexal mass and often demonstrates striking enhancement on contrast-enhanced CT or MRI [18]. Histologically, dysgerminoma is characterized by large cells with prominent centrally located nuclei and clear cytoplasm (so-called fried egg appearance). Ten to fifteen percent of patients with dysgerminoma will present with bilateral ovarian involvement and lymphatic spread can occur [19].

Dysgerminoma can develop within gonadoblastoma in patients with dysgenetic gonads. XY gonadal dysgenesis is associated with an elevated risk of developing germ cell malignancy, reported as 30–50 % in some series [20]. Girls with complete androgen insensitivity syndrome present with primary amenorrhea and may also be at increased risk for gonadoblastoma and MOGCT [21].

Endodermal sinus tumors, EST, are aggressive, MOGCT characterized by rapid growth and frequent metastasis throughout the abdomen and pelvis. AFP is a sensitive and specific marker, often in the hundred to thousand range at diagnosis, and can be used to monitor response to therapy. Imaging most often demonstrates a complex cystic and solid mass with necrosis and areas of hemorrhage [22]. Microscopically, tumors are comprised of tubules lined by flattened cuboidal cells. Rosettes of papillary tumor cells with a central vessel form the pathognomonic Schiller–Duval body [23].

Immature teratomas affect younger patients with a median age at diagnosis of 17 and represent 10–20 % of all ovarian cancers in patients under age 20 [24]. Imaging characteristics are similar to that seen in mature cystic teratoma and show a complex cystic and solid mass with areas of fat [13]. Immature teratomas are composed of tissue from all three germ layers but it is the presence of immature neural elements which confers malignant behavior. Immature teratomas are the only germ cell tumor that is histologically graded. Grade is determined by the proportion of the tumor containing immature neurologic elements [25]. Higher grade is associated with an increased risk for extraovarian spread and worse overall survival [26].

Embryonal carcinoma, polyembryoma, and nongestational choriocarcinoma are rare and aggressive MOGCTs encountered in the pediatric and adolescent population. These tumors may produce HCG which can result in isosexual precocious puberty in young girls [16].

Treatment of germ cell tumors consists of surgery followed in most cases by chemotherapy. In patients with normal chromosomes who desire future fertility, ovarian cystectomy or unilateral oophorectomy and staging should be performed.

Staging of MOGCT in children and adolescents should consist of:

1. Collection of ascites or peritoneal washings upon entry into the abdomen
2. Careful inspection and palpation of the peritoneal surfaces with biopsy or excision of any nodules
3. Inspection and palpation of the omentum with resection of any adherent or abnormal areas
4. Assessment of the pelvic and paraaortic lymph node basins with biopsy of enlarged or firm lymph nodes
5. Complete resection of the affected ovary
6. Inspection of the contralateral ovary with biopsy of any abnormal areas

Current Children's Oncology Group (COG) guidelines recommend against systematic dissection of retroperitoneal lymph nodes in children and young adolescents with apparent early stage MOGCT [27]. Biopsy of a normal appearing contralateral ovary is discouraged to avoid impairing future fertility [28]. An open approach to surgery via laparotomy is strongly encouraged in children as the current staging guidelines rely on both visual and tactile assessment of anatomic structures. This differs somewhat from management of adult women where laparoscopy is increasingly used for staging of suspected early ovarian cancers. Every effort should be made to avoid spillage of tumor contents and to remove the tumor intact.

Bilateral ovarian disease is more common with dysgerminoma and teratoma. Cystectomy and confirmation of pathology should be performed prior to bilateral salpingo-oophorectomy in young women as benign mature cystic teratoma may present as a contralateral mass to a malignant germ cell tumor. Complete tumor cytoreduction should be performed in patients presenting with evidence of bulky metastatic disease. Hysterectomy, bilateral salpingo-oophorectomy, and staging are appropriate for women who have completed childbearing only and is not the appropriate surgical managment for children or adolescents, in most cases. Women who have complete or partial Y chromosome should have both gonads removed, regardless of the age of diagnosis.

While the rarity of OGCT has precluded randomized clinical trials, a large body of evidence exists in the testicular germ cell literature to guide chemotherapy choices. The BEP regimen, bleomycin, etoposide, and cisplatin, is the preferred regimen as it has been proven to be superior to other combination chemo protocols [29]. With surgery and chemotherapy prognosis is excellent, with survival exceeding 95 % [30].

The need for adjuvant chemotherapy in children and young adolescents with MOGCT has recently been questioned. Surveillance after surgery for stage I testicular cancer is considered standard of care due to the high rate of cure with surgery alone and the success of salvage chemotherapy in patients with disease recurrence [31]. The COG evaluated this surgery-only strategy in 25 children and young adolescents with stage I MOGCT. Recurrence was identified in 12 (50 %) of patients of whom 11 were successfully salvaged with combination chemotherapy [32]. Four year overall survival was 96 % and half of patients were able to avoid chemotherapy.

Stromal Tumors of the Ovary

SCST are a heterogeneous group of tumors that arise from the non-germ, non-follicular cells of the ovary: granulosa cells, theca cells, Leydig cells, Sertoli cells, and stromal fibroblasts. Malignant ovarian sex cord stromal tumors (MOSCSTs) account for approximately 10 % of malignant ovarian tumors in the pediatric and adolescent population [33]. Granulosa tumors are the most common MOSCST, accounting for 2–5 % of ovarian cancers [34]. The majority of granulosa tumors is of the adult type and occurs primarily in perimenopausal and postmenopausal women. Juvenile granulosa cell tumors (JGCTs) are less common, accounting for only 5 % of granulosa tumors overall, but comprise the majority of granulosa tumors in children and adolescents. Patients may demonstrate isosexual pseudoprecocity as a result of tumor estrogen production, but more commonly present with abdominal pain and swelling [35]. Imaging most often demonstrates a large unilateral multiloculated mass with irregular septa [13]. Histology demonstrates diffuse sheets or nodules of eosinophilic cells with immature nuclei and abundant mitotic activity [36]. JGCT cells typically lack the characteristic nuclear grooves (coffee bean nuclei) seen in mature granulosa tumors.

The majority of JGCTs present as an encapsulated tumor confined to one ovary (stage IA). Unilateral salpingo-oophorectomy and staging result in cure rates of over 95 %. Preoperative tumor rupture, malignant ascites, and high mitotic rate appear to be poor prognostic features [37]. Patients with advanced stage disease follow a dramatically different course. While the literature consists mainly of case reports and retrospective series, stage III disease has been associated with a high rate of relapse and poor 5 year survival of 0–22 % [38]. Management of patients with extraovarian disease consists of surgical debulking of all visible tumor followed by systemic chemotherapy. Although the ideal chemotherapy regimen is not yet defined, good response rates and sustained remissions have been reported in patients treated with etoposide and platinum containing regimens [37].

Sertoli–Leydig tumors of the ovary comprise less than 0.5 % of all ovarian neoplasms in children and adolescents. They occur most often in adolescents with a median age at diagnosis of 14 [39]. Sertoli–Leydig tumors may produce androgens and result in virilization and/or irregular menses or delayed menarche. Serum testosterone, inhibin, and AFP have been reported to be elevated and may be useful as tumor markers. Sertoli–Leydig cell tumors can have a variable appearance on imaging, but most often present as a predominantly solid mass [13]. Histologically they are composed of hollow or solid tubules surrounded by a fibrous stroma [36]. The degree of histologic differentiation has prognostic implications. In one series, all patients presenting with well-differentiated SLCT followed a benign course; however, 11 % of moderately differentiated and 59 % of poorly differentiated SLCT were clinically malignant [40]. Intraoperative tumor spillage may be a poor prognostic feature [41]. Adjuvant chemotherapy is generally administered to patients with stage IC-IV disease. While evidence is lacking as to the optimal regimen, as for JGCT, an etoposide and platinum containing regimen is favored.

SLCTs have been reported in association with mutations of the *DICER1* gene. *DICER1* mutations have been associated with pleuropulmonary blastoma, familial multinodular goiter, and thyroid cancer raising concern for a familial cancer syndrome [42]. Genetic counseling should be considered for young patients with SLCT and a suggestive family history.

Uncommon Ovarian Tumors

Small cell carcinoma of the ovary hypercalcemic type, SCCOHT, is a rare and aggressive cancer affecting women under the age of 40. Patients present with abdominal pain and distension as in other malignant ovarian tumors. Hypercalcemia is present in approximately two-thirds of patients but is most often asymptomatic [43]. In the largest series reported to date, bilateral ovarian involvement was common and 50 % of patients presented with stage III and IV disease [44]. The cell of origin of SCCOHT is unknown. The histologic appearance is variable, most often consisting of sheets of homogeneous small blue cells with a high mitotic rate. Large cells with bland cytoplasm may be mixed with small cells and the differential diagnosis includes JGCT, lymphoma, metastatic small cell carcinoma of the lung, and metastatic melanoma [44]. Survival is poor regardless of stage at diagnosis and treatment consists of aggressive surgery followed by systemic chemotherapy.

Epithelial ovarian tumors are extremely rare in the pediatric and adolescent population and when present most commonly demonstrate borderline histology. Borderline tumors occur more often in older adolescents and women in the third decade of life. Imaging classically demonstrates a multicystic adnexal mass with papillary projections and mural nodularity. CA 125 may be elevated. Treatment consists of fertility preserving surgery with cystectomy or unilateral oophorectomy. Presence of extra ovarian disease increases the risk for recurrence but does not necessarily confer worse survival. Chemotherapy has not been shown to decrease the risk for recurrence and is not recommended except in those patients with metastatic disease showing invasive implants [45].

Leukemia or lymphoma can rarely metastasize to the ovary; such tumors account for less than 2 % of all pediatric ovarian

tumors [8]. Imaging demonstrates unilateral or bilateral solid
adnexal masses, often with small cysts, corresponding to preserved
follicles, in the periphery of the ovary [13].

Fertility Preservation in Children and Adolescents with Ovarian Cancer

An important goal of treatment of ovarian cancers in children and
adolescents is preservation of normal fertility potential. While
ovarian cystectomy is recommended for treatment of benign ovarian neoplasms, unilateral oophorectomy is strongly recommended
for patients diagnosed with ovarian malignancy. Importantly, ovarian function, as measured by menstrual regularity, does not appear
to be compromised by removal of one gonad [46]. No statistical
difference in long-term fertility was observed in women who had
undergone unilateral oophorectomy when compared to cohorts of
patients undergoing non-gynecologic pelvic or upper abdominal
surgery [47]. Chemotherapy, particularly exposure to high doses of
alkylating agents, may result in ovarian dysfunction [48]. Pregnancy
rates were noted to be significantly lower in women who received
more than three cycle of cisplatin-based chemotherapy for MOGCT
when compared to those who received no chemotherapy or
<3 cycles of chemotherapy [49]. Assessment of serum anti-Mülle-
rian hormone (AMH) may provide a measure of ovarian reserve in
survivors of childhood cancer [50].

  Gonadotropin-releasing hormone agonists have been evaluated
for the prevention of ovarian toxicity during chemotherapy. A recent
randomized control trial demonstrated significantly lower rates of
premature ovarian failure in reproductive age breast cancer patients
receiving goserelin and chemotherapy compared to those receiving
chemotherapy alone [51]. While not specifically studied in young
women with ovarian cancer, use of GNRH agonist therapy may be
considered in menarchal adolescents who will receive systemic chemotherapy. Young girls and women who may be at risk for cancer-
associated infertility should be offered referral to a reproductive
endocrinologist for consideration of oocyte cryopreservation [52].

Patients who receive fertility sparing treatment of malignant ovarian neoplasms in childhood and adolescence should undergo careful clinical surveillance in the years that follow. Most recurrences will occur within the first 2 years of treatment. Dysgerminomas and stromal tumors, however, are characterized by delayed recurrence, which can occur years or even decades after initial treatment. A reasonable strategy is to perform clinical exam, pelvic ultrasound, and serum tumor marker assessment at 3–4 month intervals for the first 2 years, switching to semi-annual to annual visits over the next several years. Careful attention should be directed to monitoring for signs of treatment associated toxicities such as ovarian dysfunction and secondary malignancy.

Management

Preoperative bloodwork revealed a serum testosterone of 137 and AFP of 204. All other tumor markers, including HCG, CA 125, Inhibin, and LDH, were within normal limits. The patient was taken to the operating room urgently for a presumed diagnosis of a malignant ovarian mass. Exploratory laparotomy revealed a multiloculated mass arising from the left adnexa and 0.5 L of ascites. A normal right ovary and uterus were identified. The omentum was densely adherent to the left adnexal mass. Shotty adenopathy was noted in the paraaortic nodal basins. Left salpingo-oophorectomy, omentectomy and biopsies of left pelvic and paraaortic lymph nodes was performed without complication. Pathology demonstrated a moderately differentiated Sertoli–Leydig cell tumor of the left ovary.

Outcome

Cytology and all staging biopsies were negative. The final diagnosis was of a stage IA moderately differentiated Sertoli–Leydig cell tumor. Serum testosterone and AFP normalized at 1 month after surgery. Clinical surveillance visits occur at 4 month intervals at which time testosterone and AFP are assessed. Pelvic ultrasound is obtained twice yearly. Two years after surgery she remains without evidence of disease.

Clinical Pearls and Pitfalls

1. OGCT and SCST can be associated with precocious or delayed menarche as a result of hormones produced by the tumor.
2. Precocious puberty occurs in less than 10 % of patients with childhood ovarian malignancies.
3. MOGCT may present with concurrent contralateral benign cystic teratomas. Cystectomy and histologic assessment should be performed prior to performing bilateral oophorectomy.
4. Large mass size (>10 cm) and presence of solid components are highly suggestive of malignancy. Assessment of tumor markers and surgical intervention by an appropriately trained clinician should be undertaken without delay.
5. Fertility preserving surgery with unilateral oophorectomy and surgical staging according to the COG guidelines is the appropriate approach in nearly all children and adolescents with ovarian tumors, except when obvious metastatic disease is present.
6. Ovarian malignancies in children and young women are highly curable.
7. Girls presenting with amenorrhea secondary to XY gonadal dysgenesis should undergo bilateral gonadectomy because of an associated elevated risk of developing gonadoblastoma and other germ cell malignancies in the dysgenetic gonads.

References

1. Skinner MA, Schlatter MG, et al. Ovarian neoplasms in children. Arch Surg. 1993;128(8):849–53.
2. Diamond MP, Baxter JW, et al. Occurrence of ovarian malignancies in childhood and adolescence; a community-wide evaluation. Obstet Gynecol. 1988;71(6 Pt 1):858–60.

3. Merino MJ, Jaffe G. Age contrast in ovarian pathology. Cancer. 1993;71 (2 suppl):537–44.

4. Oltmann SC, Garcia N, et al. Can we preoperatively risk stratify ovarian masses for malignancy? J Pediatr Surg. 2010;45(1):130–4.

5. Schultz KA, Sencer SF, et al. Pediatric ovarian tumors: a review of 67 cases. Pediatr Blood Cancer. 2005;44(2):167–73.

6. Papic JC, Finnell SM, et al. Predictors of ovarian malignancy in children: overcoming clinical barriers of ovarian preservation. J Pediatr Surg. 2014; 49(1):144–7.

7. Oltmann SC, Garcia NM, et al. Pediatric ovarian malignancies: how efficacious are current staging practices? J Pediatr Surg. 2010;45(6):1096–102.

8. Oltmann SC, Fischer A, et al. Pediatric ovarian malignancies presenting as ovarian torsion: incidence and relevance. J Pediatr Surg. 2010; 45(1):135–9.

9. Cass DL, Hawkins E, et al. Surgery for ovarian masses in infants, children, and adolescents: 102 consecutive patients treated in a 15-year period. J Pediatr Surg. 2001;36(5):693–9.

10. Mashiach R, Melamed N, et al. Sonographic diagnosis of ovarian torsion: accuracy and predictive factors. J Ultrasound Med. 2011;30(9):1205–10.

11. Wilkinson C, Sanderson A. Adnexal torsion—a multimodality imaging review. Clin Radiol. 2012;67(5):476–83.

12. Young Jr JL, Cheng Wu X, et al. Ovarian cancer in children and young adults in the United States, 1992-1997. Cancer. 2003;97(10 suppl): 2694–700.

13. Heo SH, Kim JW, et al. Review of ovarian tumors in children and adolescents: radiologic-pathologic correlation. Radiographics. 2014;34(7): 2039–55.

14. Mann AP, Grebenciucova E, et al. Anti-N-methyl-D-aspartate-receptor encephalitis: diagnosis, optimal management and challenges. Ther Risk Manage. 2014;10:517–25.

15. Smith HO, Berwick M, et al. Incidence and survival rates for female malignant germ cell tumors. Obstet Gynecol. 2006;107(5):1075–85.

16. Abu-Rustum NR, Aghajanian C. Management of malignant germ cell tumors of the ovary. Semin Oncol. 1998;25(2):235–42.

17. Young Jr JL, Miller RW. Incidence of malignant tumors in U.S. children. J Pediatr. 1975;86:254–8.

18. Tanaka YO, Kurosaki Y, et al. Ovarian dysgerminoma: MR and CT appearance. J Comput Assist Tomogr. 1994;18(3):443–8.

19. Boran N, Tulunay G, et al. Pregnancy outcomes and menstrual function after fertility sparing surgery for pure ovarian dysgerminomas. Arch Gynecol Obstet. 2005;271(2):104–8.

20. Hanlon AJ, Kimble RM. Incidental gonadal tumors at the time of gonadectomy in women with Swyer syndrome: a case series. J Pediatr Adolesc Gynecol. 2014;28(2):e27–9.

21. Levin H. Tumors of the testis in intersex syndromes. Urol Clin North Am. 2000;27(3):543–51.

22. Levitin A, Haller KD, et al. Endodermal sinus tumors of the ovary: imaging evaluations. AJR Am J Roentgenol. 1996;167(3):791–3.
23. Talerman A. Germ cell tumours of the ovary. In: Kurman RJ, editor. Blaustein's pathology of the female genital tract. New York: Springer; 1994. p. 849.
24. Gershenson DM, del Junco G, et al. Immature teratoma of the ovary. Obstet Gynecol. 1986;68(5):624–9.
25. Norris HJ, Zirkin HJ, et al. Immature (malignant) teratoma of the ovary: a clinical and pathologic study of 58 cases. Cancer. 1976;37(5):2359–72.
26. O'Connor DM, Norris HJ. The influence of grade on the outcome of stage I ovarian immature (malignant) teratomas and the reproducibility of grading. Int J Gynecol Pathol. 1994;13(4):283–9.
27. Billmire D, Vinocur C. Outcome and staging evaluation in malignant germ cell tumors of the ovary in children and adolescents: an intergroup study. J Pediatr Surg. 2004;39(3):424–9.
28. Pectasides D, Pectasides E, et al. Germ cell tumors of the ovary. Cancer Treat Rev. 2008;34(5):427–41.
29. Cushing B, Giller R, et al. Randomized comparison of combination chemotherapy with etoposide, bleomycin and either high-dose or standard-dose cisplatin in children and adolescents with high-risk malignant germ cell tumors: a pediatric intergroup study. J Clin Oncol. 2004;22(13): 2691–700.
30. Park JY, Kim DY, et al. Outcomes of pediatric and adolescent girls with malignancy ovarian germ cell tumors. Gynecol Oncol. 2015;137(3):418–22. doi:10.1016/j.ygyno.2015.03.054.
31. Schlatter M, Rescorla F, et al. Excellent outcome in patients with stage I germ cell tumors of the testes: a study of the Children's Oncology Group/ Pediatric Oncology Group. J Pediatr Surg. 2003;38(3):319–24.
32. Billmire DF, Cullen JW, et al. Surveillance after initial surgery for pediatric and adolescent girls with stage I ovarian germ cell tumors: report from the Children's Oncology Group. J Clin Oncol. 2014;32(5):465–70.
33. Schneider DT, Terenziani M. Gonadal and extragonadal germ cell tumors, sex cord stromal tumors and rare gonadal tumors. In: Brecht IB, editor. Rare tumors in children and adolescents. Heidelberg: Springer; 2012. p. 327–402.
34. Young RH. Sex cord-stromal tumors of the ovary and testis: their similarities and differences with consideration of selected problems. Mod Pathol. 2005;18 suppl 2:S81–98.
35. Cecchetto G, Ferrari A, et al. Sex cord stromal tumors of the ovary in children: a clinicopathological report from the Italian TREP project. Pediatr Blood Cancer. 2011;56(7):1062–7.
36. Young R. Ovarian tumors and tumor-like lesions in the first three decades. Semin Pathol. 2014;31(5):382–426.
37. Schneider DT, Calaminus G, et al. Ovarian sex cord-stromal tumors in children and adolescents. J Clin Oncol. 2003;21(12):2357–63.

38. Powell JL, Kotwall CA, et al. Fertility-sparing surgery for advanced juvenile granulosa cell tumor of the ovary. J Pediatr Adolesc Gynecol. 2014; 27(4):e89–92.
39. Schneider DT, Jänig U, et al. Ovarian sex cord-stromal tumors: a clinicopathologic study of 72 cases from the Kiel Pediatric Tumor Registry. Virchows Arch. 2003;443(4):549–60.
40. Young RH, Scully RE. Ovarian Sertoli-Leydig cell tumors. A clinicopathological analysis of 207 cases. Am J Surg Pathol. 1985;9(8):543–69.
41. Schneider DT, Orbach D, et al. Ovarian Sertoli Leydig cell tumours in children and adolescents: an analysis of the European Cooperative Study Group on Pediatric Rare Tumors (EXPeRT). Eur J Cancer. 2015; 51(4):543–50.
42. Schultze-Florey RE, Graf N, et al. DICER1 syndrome: a new cancer syndrome. Klin Padiatr. 2013;225(3):177–8.
43. Zaied S, Gharbi O, et al. Small cell carcinoma of the ovary of hypercalcemic type: a case report. Case Rep Oncol Med. 2012;2012:461873.
44. Young RH, Oliva E, et al. Small cell carcinoma of the ovary, hypercalcemic type: a clinicopathologic analysis of 150 cases. Am J Surg Pathol. 1994;18(11):1102–16.
45. NIH consensus conference. Ovarian cancer. Screening, treatment, and follow-up. NIH Consensus Development Panel on Ovarian Cancer. JAMA. 1995;273(6):491–7.
46. Zhai A, Axt J, et al. Assessing gonadal function after childhood ovarian surgery. J Pediatr Surg. 2012;47(6):1272–9.
47. Bellati F, Ruscito I. Effects of unilateral ovariectomy on female fertility outcomes. Arch Gynecol Obstet. 2014;290(2):349–53.
48. Schilsky RL, Lewis BJ, et al. Gonadal dysfunction in patients receiving chemotherapy for cancer. Ann Intern Med. 1980;93(1):109–14.
49. Solheim O, Tropé CG, et al. Fertility and gonadal function after adjuvant therapy in women diagnosed with a malignant ovarian germ cell tumor (MOGCT) during the "cisplatin era". Gynecol Oncol. 2013;136(2):224–9.
50. Lunsford AJ, Whelan K, et al. Antimullerian hormone as a measure of reproductive function in female childhood cancer survivors. Fertil Steril. 2014;101(1):227–31.
51. Moore HC, Unger JM, et al. Goserelin for ovarian protection during breast-cancer adjuvant chemotherapy. N Engl J Med. 2015;372(23):2269–70.
52. ACOG. Gynecologic concerns in children and adolescents with cancer. Committee Opinion No. 607. Obset Gynecol. 2014;124(2 Pt 1):403–8.

Chapter 12
Survivors of Childhood Cancer and Cancer Treatments

May-Tal Sauerbrun-Cutler, Christine Mullin, and Avner Hershlag

Abbreviations

ABVD	Doxorubicin, bleomycin, vinblastine, dacarbazine
AML	Acute myelocytic anemia
ART	Advanced reproductive technology
BMT	Bone marrow transplant
CNS	Central nervous system
CSI	Cranial spinal irradiation
FSH	Follicle-stimulating hormone
GH	Growth hormone
ICSI	Intra-cytoplasmic sperm Injection
IVM	In vitro maturation
LH	Luteinizing hormone
MOPP	Mechlorethamine, vincristine, procarbazine, prednisone
POF	Premature ovarian failure
TBR	Total body radiation

M.-T. Sauerbrun-Cutler, M.D. • C. Mullin, M.D.
A. Hershlag, M.D. (✉)
Center for Human Reproduction, North Shore University Hospital—LIJ,
Hofstra University School of Medicine, 300 Community Drive,
Manhasset, NY 11030, USA
e-mail: Hershla@nshs.edu

© Springer International Publishing Switzerland 2016
H.L. Appelbaum (ed.), *Abnormal Female Puberty*,
DOI 10.1007/978-3-319-27225-2_12

Introduction

As survival of childhood cancer continues to increase, it is incumbent upon us to pay closer attention to the quality of life of children and adolescents, understand the potential risks of aggressive treatment to the normal pubertal development, and develop an algorithm that affords the best possible reproductive outcome.

According to the National Cancer Registry, there were 55,486 female childhood and adolescent cancer cases during 2001–2009, with an age-adjusted incidence rate of 161.96 per million. The three most common malignancies identified were leukemia, CNS malignancy, and lymphoma (41, 29, 21 per 1,000,000 females aged 0–19, respectively) [1]. Radiation and chemotherapy pose risks to pubertal development and fertility potential. Chemotherapy and radiation therapy may result in arrested or delayed puberty and survivors have a 35 % risk of developing an endocrine disorder by age 40 [2]. Cranial radiation is a common treatment for leukemia, lymphoma, and brain malignancy which leads to both precocious puberty and pituitary hormone deficiencies. Growth hormone (GH) deficiency is the most common disorder in brain cancer survivors. Gonadotropin hormone deficiency may occur at exposures to over 30 Gy [3, 4]. Pelvic or whole body radiation can cause permanent ovarian failure and pubertal arrest at doses of 20 Gy or greater. Even if ovarian function and menses are maintained, women are still at risk for pregnancy-related complications and premature ovarian insufficiency. Chemotherapy is not as harmful as radiation because it is less likely to cause permanent amenorrhea. However, chemotherapy combined with radiation therapy, as well as high dose alkylating agents alone, frequently leads to cessation of pubertal development and/or premature ovarian failure (POF). Hormone replacement therapy (HRT) is critical to induce development of sexual characteristics in patients with pubertal dysfunction. Estrogen therapy is the initial treatment followed by addition of progesterone after breast development commences. Consultation, prior to oncologic treatment, regarding fertility preservation is imperative as successful oocyte and embryo cryopreservation are established techniques with high success rates. Prepubertal patients do not have eggs to freeze and the only option is ovarian tissue cryopreservation with transplantation in later life. A recent reported success of this approach makes it an exciting option as more experience is gained. Ovarian transposition out of the field of radiation has a moderate success rate and should be considered for patients undergoing abdominal surgery and adjuvant pelvic irradiation.

Case Presentation 1

A 16-year-old female is referred to the endocrinologist for primary amenorrhea. She complains of lethargy, 10 lb weight gain, and cold intolerance. Her medical history is significant for Hodgkin disease (HD) stage IV B at age 11 treated with MOPP, ABVD, and total body radiation (TBR). Subsequently, she developed AML at age 13 and was treated with a bone marrow transplant (BMT).

On exam, she weighs 130 lb and is 60 in. There is no thyromegaly. She has Tanner stage 5 breast and pubic hair development. Pelvic exam reveals normal external genitalia. The vagina is normal in length and caliber. The uterus is palpable below the pubic bone and the ovaries are nonpalpable.

Lab tests are significant for elevated TSH and low free T4. Prolactin, luteinizing hormone (LH), follicle-stimulating hormone (FSH), estradiol, growth hormone (GH), DHEA-sulfate (DHEAS), and testosterone are all normal. Pelvic ultrasound reveals normal size ovaries, 7 week size uterus with 6 mm endometrial stripe.

Discussion

The patient is experiencing primary amenorrhea secondary to the chemotherapy and TBR she received, first for the Hodgkin disease, then in preparation for BMT. While she still managed to produce enough estrogen to develop secondary sexual characteristics, she hasn't managed to make estrogen above the threshold level required for menarche.

Children and adolescents exposed to toxic cancer treatments have a better prognosis for preservation of reproductive function than older women [5, 8]. Nevertheless, Primordial and developing follicles are sensitive to radiation, which may lead to follicular atresia as well as cortical atrophy in children exposed to high dose radiation. The effective sterilizing dose causing permanent POF is age-dependent as seen in Table 12.1 [5]. Permanent ovarian failure and subsequently pubertal arrest occur in childhood cancers treated with ovarian radiation doses more than 20 Gy [6]. The dose of fractionated radiation therapy at which ovarian failure occurs immediately after treatment in 97.5 % of females (also known as the "effective sterilizing dose") is 20.3 Gy (divided into 1.5–2.0 Gy fractions) at birth and decreases to 16.5 Gy at age 20 years [7]. However, the median lethal dose (the dose needed to decrease the ovarian follicular pool by 50 %) is as low as 2 Gy [7].

At the time of the radiation exposure, this patient was in early puberty. Furthermore, the patient has signs and symptoms of hypothyroidism which likely occurred after radiation exposure to the thyroid. Radiation therapy to the neck (for Hodgkin lymphoma (HL), brain tumors, head and neck sarcomas, and acute lymphoblastic leukemia) may result in hypothyroidism in as many as 33–50 % of patients who receive doses of >35 Gy [9]. If not properly treated, thyroid disease may be a culprit in delayed maturation and poor linear growth [10]. Radiation therapy exhibits a clear dose-related toxicity to the thyroid gland, with a 20-year risk of hypothyroidism of 20 % at <35 Gy, 30 % at 35–44.9 Gy, and 50 % at >45 Gy to the neck [11]. On average, thyroid dysfunction develops 2–5 years posttreatment.

The chemotherapy regimen this patient received was ABVD and MOPP. ABVD is considered less gonadotoxic than MOPP since MOPP contains the alkylating agent procarbazine [12]. The extent of ovarian damage after chemotherapy treatment is influenced by type of drug administered, dosage, and the age of patient at treatment. Alkylating agents cause the highest risk of POF because they damage DNA and induce apoptosis through binding

Table 12.1 Effective sterilizing dose [8]

At birth	20.3 Gy
10 years	18.4 Gy
20 years	16.5 Gy
30 years	14.3 Gy

of alkyl groups to DNA. Other common alkylating agents include cyclophosphamide and busulfan. Alkylating agents are cell cycle nonspecific, therefore they can damage even resting oocytes [13]. Meirow et al. studied different cancers in 168 females aged 13–40 [13] indicating odds ratios for different chemotherapy agents for causing ovarian failure defined as amenorrhea and/or elevated levels of gonadotropins present at least 6 months after completion of chemotherapy treatment. Patients treated by drugs of the alkylating agents group had a 42.4 % ovarian failure rate, the highest of any chemotherapy agent. Studies show that even if cyclophosphamide caused immediate amenorrhea, the effects were reversible in >50 % of adolescents by 3–42 months in many studies [14]. Cessation of menses occurs as a result of the destruction of growing follicles. Recovery of ovarian function is common for most female childhood cancer patients treated initially with combination chemotherapy and most resume menses unless given adjuvant radiation or dose intensive alkylating agents for myeloablative conditioning before stem cell transplant. Table 12.2 provides a list of the gonadotoxicity of different classes of chemotherapeutic agents.

BMT survivors such as this patient have the most severe gonadal damage. Most of these patients are preconditioned with high doses of chemotherapeutic agents and total body radiation. A retrospective cohort study of 92 survivors of allogeneic HSCT at childhood <20 years of age evaluated long-term ovarian function after allogeneic hematopoietic stem cell transplantation (SCT) [20]. Only 50 % of Leukemia patients (ALL and AML) had achieved spontaneous puberty and 30 % spontaneous menarche at their latest follow-up visit. Similar results were found in a single center cohort study of 109 women with transplants during childhood where the cumulative incidence of ovarian insufficiency (OI) was 56 % at a median follow-up of 7.2 years. Forty five percent had ovarian insufficiency if the HSCT was performed in the prepubertal age group, 67 % during puberty, and 79 % postpubertal ($P<0.001$) [21].

It is unclear whether the patient will begin menstruating, however; normal FSH and estradiol levels are encouraging. Childhood cancer survivors treated with doses of radiation >30 Gy to the hypothalamic–pituitary axis are at risk for LH and FSH deficiency causing hypothalamic amenorrhea. Her normal FSH and LH indicate that she does not have central or hypothalamic amenorrhea.

Table 12.2 Gonadotoxicity of chemotherapeutic agents

Chemotherapy class	Chemotherapy agent	Level of gonadotoxicity
Alkylating	Cyclophosphamide, Melphalan	High toxicity [15, 16]
	Chlorambucil, Busulfan	
	Nitrogen mustard	
Platinum	Cisplatin, Carboplatin	Moderate toxicity [17]
Antibiotics	Anthracycline family: Doxorubicin	Moderate toxicity [18]
Plant alkaloids	Taxane: Paclitaxel	Moderate Toxicity
• Spindle Poisons mitotic inhibitor	Vinca: Vinblastine, Vincristine	
Antibiotics	Streptomyces: Actinomycin	Mild toxicity [18]
Antimetabolites	Folic acid: Methotrexate, Aminopertin	Mild toxicity [15, 17, 19]
	Purine: Mercaptopurine	
	Pyrimidine: Fluorouracil	
Plant alkaloids	Topotecan	Unknown
• Topoisomerase inhibitors	Etoposide, Teniposide	

Management

Given the wide range of reported incidence of pubertal disruption in pediatric cancer survivors, careful screening, follow-up, and early intervention are essential to help these girls achieve their pubertal milestones. The Children's Oncology Group recommends screening girls who received alkylating agents or pelvic radiation with serum gonadotropins (FSH and LH) by age 13 [22]. Normal level warrants repeat levels in 6 months. An overall assessment of ovarian reserve is important. Some patients with normal FSH and LH may still have low ovarian reserve and a shortened reproductive life span. While ovarian reserve markers such as anti-mullerian hormone (AMH), FSH, Inhibin B, and antral follicle count (AFC) have been used, none have been validated as standard of care for young patients. Some studies have shown that AMH is better than FSH especially for prepubertal patients [23]. AMH is produced in the granulosa cells in late preantral and small antral follicles. AMH participates in the regulation of oocyte development from the primordial follicle pool, setting the pace at which follicles reenter meiosis and thus the rate of depletion of the primordial follicle pool [24]. Blood levels have been used to attempt to measure the size of the pool of growing follicles in women. It has become one of the most widely used markers in adult patients as part of the infertility evaluation; however, its levels in adolescents have not been widely studied. FSH is less reliable than AMH because of its intra-cycle variability and also it can be falsely low due to a quiescent hypothalamic–pituitary–ovarian axis in prepubertal children, use of OCPs, or in patients who developed central hypogonadotropic hypogonadism.

If this patient's menses do not begin, or her FSH values increase into postmenopausal range, then HRT should be recommended. Replacement therapy with estrogen and progesterone may be necessary to provide secondary sexual development and induce or maintain puberty including the development of breast tissue, attainment of appropriate stature, induction of menses, growth of the uterus for possible reproductive function, and maintenance of skeletal health [25]. In addition, hormonal replacement improves long-term quality of life for girls with ovarian failure who have already completed the pubertal process. Despite these benefits, the optimal HRT regimen is unclear as data in adolescents is limited.

Estrogen therapy is usually started by age 12–13 and must be prescribed and monitored by a pediatric endocrinologist, aiming to induce development of secondary sexual characteristics, achieve an acceptable final height, and maintain bone density. If administered incorrectly, there is a risk of premature closure of the epiphysis [21, 26]. Data has shown that if therapy is started at 12 years old with low doses, there is no detrimental effect on height [25]. DiVasta and Gordon advise giving HRT in three phases [27]:

- *Phase 1*: Induction of breast development: Only low dose estrogen is given to stimulate breast development in an adolescent who lacks signs of secondary sexual development in order to replicate early puberty where progesterone does not play a role. The starting dose is 1/8th–1/10th of an adult dose or 5 mg/kg body weight/day. Estrogen can be administered orally or via transdermal route. Some examples of common starting doses are as follows: conjugated equine estrogen 0.3 mg, micronized estradiol 0.5 mg, Estraderm 25 μg transdermal patch.

- *Phase 2*: Further breast development, establishing menses, and promoting bone mineral acquisition occur 6–18 months after phase I, similar to the timing of increased hormones in spontaneous puberty. The timing depends on breast development. The following are increased doses of estrogens that are typically given: conjugated equine estrogens 0.625 mg, estrone sulfate 0.625 mg, micronized estradiol 1 mg, 50 μg transdermal estrogen patch. Cyclic progestin is added after 12–24 months of estrogen-only treatment and should be started prior to menses. Progesterone is added to protect the endometrium from the hyperplastic effects of unopposed estrogen. Available progestins include medroxyprogesterone 5–10 mg daily or micronized progesterone 200 mg daily for 5 days. Once breast development is complete, the progestin can be increased to 10 days each month. During this phase the adolescent should complete breast development and start menstruating.
- *Phase 3*: Maintenance phase progestins are usually given for 12–14 days each month to fully induce a secretory endometrium and protect against endometrial cancer, or combination products such as estrogen–progestin oral contraceptive pill (OCP), transvaginal, and transdermal preparations can be given. During this phase, higher amounts of estrogen are necessary (serum levels of approximately 100 pg/mL)

This patient has already reached Tanner stage 5. Therefore, if she needs HRT, she would go straight to Phase 3 or placed on one of the aforementioned maintenance therapy combinations.

Advantages of estrogen administration in adolescence include a higher peak bone mass and positive effect on various tissues such as the brain and cardiovascular system as well as other health endpoints such as lipid profile [28]. Contrary to recent data for menopausal women, there is evidence of significant endothelial dysfunction and cardiovascular disease for young women with premature ovarian insufficiency with no hormone repletion. Within 6 months of initiating HRT, these abnormalities resolve [28]. However, there are some potential, rare, negative effects, such as an increased risk of thrombotic events and hypertriglyceridemia.

The preferred route of maintenance HRT in adolescents is currently under debate. It is unclear whether the transdermal or oral routes are better. In case-control studies of postmenopausal women, transdermal estradiol has been associated with a lower risk of venous thromboembolism than oral estrogen [29, 30]. Whereas oral estrogens can increase thrombin generation and induce a resistance to activated protein C, causing higher coagulation profile, transdermal estrogens have minimal effects on hemostatic variables [31]. Many of the studies are flawed because they compare oral conjugated estrogens with transdermal 17b-estradiol, which is not an equivalent comparison. Nevertheless, many pediatric endocrinologists prefer prescribing the transdermal preparations over the oral pills.

Although data from randomized, controlled trials are lacking, most experts agree that physiologic estrogen and progestin replacement should be continued until patients reach 51 years, the average age of menopause in the general population [32].

Outcome

This patient began menstruating therefore she did not need HRT. However, her AMH levels were extremely low, indicating poor ovarian reserve. At the age of 26, she presented in POF with cessation of menses and FSH levels in the postmenopausal range. She was placed on a transdermal combination hormone. She will be counseled regarding fertility options, including oocyte donation and adoption.

Clinical Pearls and Pitfalls

- Amenorrhea following treatment with to chemotherapy or radiation occurs secondary to depletion of ovarian follicles
- Alkylating agents cause the highest risk of POF
- Permanent ovarian failure and pubertal arrest occur in childhood cancer treated with ovarian radiation doses more than 20 Gy
- Recovery of ovarian function and resumption of menses occur in the majority of adolescents treated with chemotherapy unless treated in combination with radiation

• HRT should be given to adolescents with delayed or arrested puberty or those who have completed pubertal development but experience POF

Case Presentation 2

A 7-year-old Caucasian female is referred for evaluation of precocious puberty. Breast development as well as pubic hair growth began at age 7. She was diagnosed with Medulloblastoma (MB) and had cranial spinal radiation at age 4. She was also treated with a chemotherapy regimen of vincristine, CCNU (Lomustine), and cisplatin.

On exam she is 80th percentile for height and 50th percentile for weight. She is Tanner stage 3 for breasts and pubic hair. External genital exam is normal. Bone age of her right hand is advanced by 1.5 years. Laboratory test included a borderline elevated LH with an elevated response to GnRH stimulation test. Her brain MRI is normal.

Discussion

This patient has central precocious puberty caused by brain radiation. Indications for work-up and treatment of precocious puberty are breast and/or pubic hair development at age 7 in Caucasian girls, and 6 in African American girls. This patient's Tanner stage is also advanced for her age. She has central or gonadotropin-dependent precocious puberty because of her elevated LH levels and positive GnRH stimulation test.

Central precocious puberty results from premature activation of the hypothalamic–pituitary–gonadal axis and subsequent early elevation of LH and FSH levels from radiation. The mechanism of the hypothalamic disinhibition that causes these premature elevations in gonadotropins is unclear. Childhood cancer survivors treated with cranial irradiation (>18 Gy) are at risk for development of central precocious puberty. The risk increases with younger age at radiation, contrary to radiation-induced hypogonadism, where the risk decreases with younger age at radiation [33]. Historically, precocious puberty has been defined as any sign of secondary sexual maturity before age 8 in girls. Girls who develop breast buds and/or pubic hair before age 8 warrant an evaluation for precocious puberty [34]. This may lead to early menarche, defined by the onset of menstrual cycles prior to 9 years and advancement of bone age >2 standard deviations for chronological age. The Children Oncology Group long-term guidelines recommend referral to an endocrinologist with Tanner staging every 6 months. LH, FSH, and bone age should be tested as well as a GnRH-stimulating test to assess for peak LH levels if baseline LH is nondiagnostic.

Management

In addition to the emotional challenges and social embarrassment experienced by girls with precocious puberty, rapid bone growth puts them at risk for short stature as adults. Premature epiphyseal fusion shortens the growth period and decreases peak height velocities during the pubertal growth spurt [35, 36]. Therefore, treatment with long acting GnRH agonist is recommended to suppress the hypothalamic–pituitary axis and improve final height. GnRH agonists are usually administered until the average age of puberty, 8–9 years in African American girls and 10 in Caucasian girls [37].

In addition, the patient may need repeat radiation and chemotherapy if she relapses and therefore a discussion at this time about fertility preservation is important as high doses of radiation and chemotherapy place this patient at high risk for acute ovarian failure. Interventions to preserve ovarian function include ovarian transposition for patients prior to pelvic radiation as well as advanced reproductive technologies (ART) such as embryo and oocyte cryopreservation.

The oophoropexy procedure, or ovarian transposition, involves moving the ovaries out of the radiation field. The procedure can be done laparoscopically or via laparotomy. It should also be recommended at the time of an abdominal surgery for malignancy where radiation therapy is anticipated. A review of laparoscopic ovarian transposition cases in 46 women <40 years old reported preserved ovarian function in 88.6 % of cases [38]. Kuohung et al. also evaluated unilateral oophoropexy before cranial spinal irradiation (CSI) in a retrospective study comparing ovarian function in 15 patients who had oophoropexy compared to 11 patients with CSI alone. There was a trend toward reduced ovarian dysfunction, defined as elevated FSH or persistent amenorrhea, in controls vs. patients treated with oophoropexy (45 % vs. 13 %, $p=0.09$) [39]. While ovarian transposition may decrease the risk of ovarian failure, efficacy varies widely and there are limited studies especially in the pediatric population [40]. Most case series and case reports describe the treatment and outcomes of adult women with limited reports in young patients. The reason for variation in success rates depends on the vascular compromise of the ovary, whether chemotherapy is used, and the dose and location of the radiation [5]. Anderson et al. reported painful ovaurian cysts in 9 of 51 patinets (17.5%) resulting in oophorectomy years after the procedure [41]. Even though most reports describe the procedure as safe, patients should be counseled regarding intraoperative and postoperative complications, as well as rare long-term sequelae such as chronic cyst formation, chronic ovarian pain, and fallopian tube infarction [5, 42].

The technique involves dissecting the ovary and fallopian tube off the uterus and suturing them to the peritoneum in a location that avoids the planned field of radiation. For example, in a cohort of girls who were about to undergo CSI for a brain tumor, Laufer et al. describe the technique where the ovary to be moved was mobilized by division of the ipsilateral utero-ovarian ligament and fallopian tube [39]. The fallopian tube on the same side was sacrificed, therefore assisted reproductive technologies (ART) are required when the only remaining functional ovary is the transposed ovary. The infundibulopelvic ligament was skeletonized to allow the ovary to be moved to the lowest point in the pelvis, and nonabsorbable silk sutures were placed to attach the ovary to the uterosacral ligaments. Alternatively, the fallopian tube can be preserved and the ovaries can be transposed as high and laterally as possible, above the pelvic brim [40]. Both the transposed and non-transposed ovaries should be marked with titanium clips to aid in localization on radiation planning films [39].

BMT patients, patients receiving abdominal radiation or receiving high dose chemotherapy, or those with relapse of disease are candidates for fertility preservation with ART. Young patients who relapse generally have enough follicles in the ovary even after chemotherapy to benefit from ART [43]. Table 12.3 describes the different fertility options available.

Table 12.3 Fertility preservation options

Method	Age group	Mode of obtaining pregnancy in future	Concerns with method
Cryopreservation of oocytes	Adult women/ postpubertal girls	Egg thaw; sperm injection (ICSI); embryo transfer to patient or surrogate	Delay in cancer treatment
			Hormone injections
Cryopreservation of embryos	Adult women/ postpubertal girls	Thaw embryos; transfer to patient or surrogate	Delay in cancer treatment Hormone injections
			Availability of partner or sperm donor
Cryopreservation of ovarian tissue	Adult women/ postpubertal girls/ prepubertal girls	Reimplantation (heterotopic or orthotopic) to patient with spontaneous conception or IVF	Potential reintroduction of cancer cells
			Considered experimental

Premenarche

Cryopreservation of ovarian tissue or direct transplantation is the most appropriate method for fertility preservation in young patients. An ovary or part of ovary is removed surgically usually in a minimally invasive approach and the cortex is isolated and frozen with cryoprotectant. Meirow et al. demonstrated that laparoscopic ovarian tissue collection could be safely performed at short notice and did not delay chemotherapy, in a prospective study on 45 young cancer patients and 20 volunteers [13]. In cases where sterilization is highly likely such as in BMT, unilateral oophorectomy for cryopreservation can be performed instead of taking biopsies with a biopter. The process of vitrification is the most successful type of cryopreservation which uses a high concentration >40 % DMSO or PROH and exposes the tissue at 0 °C subsequently transferring it into liquid nitrogen. The tissue immediately turns to a glasslike state, with no crystal formation. The cortex contains the primordial follicles and is cut into 1–2 mm strips prior to cryopreservation. Once the patient is disease free these cortical strips can be reimplanted with hopes of spontaneous menses/ovulation and pregnancy. Alternatively, once the patient is ready for pregnancy the cryopreserved strips can be thawed and matured in vitro (IVM) with subsequent IVF and ICSI. Both techniques are considered experimental (either reimplantation of thawed slices of ovarian cortex or IVM from cryopreserved ovarian tissue).

There is also a theoretical risk of reintroducing malignant cells with the ovarian tissue when reimplanting pieces of ovarian cortex back to the patient [44]. Therefore, it is important to test tissue before transferring it back to the patient via histochemical staining and PCR if the disease has known genetic markers. Leukemia poses a special risk of reintroducing disease with the transplantation of tissue [5]. The most concerning conditions are the leukemias, as well as Burkitt's lymphoma and neuroblastoma. In Hodgkin lymphoma, occult tumor in ovarian pieces is rare.

In a molecular study of biopsied ovarian tissue by quantitative RT-PCR, 2 of 6 CML patients were positive for BCR-ABL mutations in their ovarian tissue. Among the 12 ALL patients, 7 of the 10 with available molecular markers showed positive leukemic markers in their ovarian tissue (translocations or rearrangement genes). In an animal model, four mice grafted with ovarian tissue from ALL patients developed intraperitoneal leukemic masses. Therefore, it is safest to offer this technique to girls with non-ovarian, non-hematologic cancers, while for patients with ALL and AML only offer it after their initial chemotherapy is completed.

Several centers have specialized in cryopreservation of ovarian tissue. For example, in the Netherlands, one center has cryopreserved over 350 samples from cancer patients with 24 % of them younger than 18 years of age [43]. Although this technique is considered experimental, it has been widely performed at many centers worldwide and is the only fertility preservation technique that can be offered rapidly to prepubertal children.

There are two main approaches for autotransplantation of human ovarian tissue [45–47]. In heterotopic transplantation, cortical fragments can be grafted subcutaneously at various sites, whereas in orthotopic transplantation cortical pieces are transplanted into their original location. Orthotopic transplantation has had more success than heterotopic transplantation. Recently, the first live birth after orthotopic transplantation of ovarian tissue harvested before menarche was reported in a women with primary ovarian failure after a myeloablative conditioning regimen as part of a hematopoietic SCT performed for homozygous sickle cell anemia at age 14 years [48]. However, the advantage of heterotopic transplantation is that it does not require general anesthesia or abdominal surgery. Various body sites can be used to graft ovarian pieces: subcutaneous space above the brachioradialis fascia of the forearm or under rectus sheet in the lower abdomen. Heterotopic transplantation may be indicated if the pelvis is not suitable for transplantation due to previous radiation or severe scar formation. There are still numerous challenges to perfecting the heterotopic ovarian transplants as the oocyte maturation process is altered compared to the orthotopic environment.

Post-menarche

Hormone stimulation with cryopreservation of oocytes or embryos is a viable option for postmenarchal girls. Results of thawing and replacing frozen embryos are excellent with pregnancy rates now over 50 %. However, feasibility is limited because embryo cryopreservation may be unrealistic for young adolescents who do not have long-term partners. Oocyte cryopreservation is an option for adolescents without partners. Pregnancy rates are progressively improving given the advances in cryopreservation technology. Some centers have reported birthrates >50 % among young patients with a live birthrate of 5–15 % mature oocyte retrieved [49].

The challenge of oocyte or embryo cryopreservation is the short window of opportunity to stimulate the ovaries, given the urgency to start cancer treatment as soon as possible. Stimulation protocols have been modified successfully to start anytime in the cycle, including the luteal phase, thus shortening the process to no longer than 2 weeks [50].

Outcomes

This patient was placed on a GnRH agonist and her pubertal development was monitored every 4–6 months with no further pubertal progression. Her parents will consider oocyte cryopreservation once she begins menstruating because she is at risk for cancer relapse and may need further treatments that could potentially further compromise ovarian function.

Clinical Pearls/Pitfalls

- Indications for a precocious puberty evaluation include breast or pubic hair development at age 7 in Caucasian girls and 6 in African American girls.
- Evaluation for precocious puberty includes Tanner staging and evaluation of gonadotropins and bone age. A GnRH-stimulating test may be indicated to assess for peak LH levels if baseline LH is nondiagnostic.
- Oophoropexy surgery or ovarian transposition involves moving the ovaries out of radiation field. It may be offered prior to radiation or before more intensive treatments especially when a patient is already scheduled for abdominal surgery.

- There are three different types of ART available for adolescents depending on their pubertal stage: Cryopreservation of ovarian tissue, oocytes, or embryos. Cryopreservation of ovarian tissue is still considered experimental and is the only option for pre-pubertal girls.

References

1. Siegel DA et al. Cancer incidence rates and trends among children and adolescents in the United States, 2001–2009. Pediatrics. 2014;134(4):e945–55.
2. de Fine Licht S et al. Hospital contacts for endocrine disorders in Adult Life after Childhood Cancer in Scandinavia (ALiCCS): a population-based cohort study. Lancet. 2014;383(9933):1981–9.
3. Sklar, Friedman, Poplack. Endocrinopathies in childhood survivors. 2014.
4. Sklar CA, Constine LS. Chronic neuroendocrinological sequelae of radiation therapy. Int J Radiat Oncol Biol Phys. 1995;31(5):1113–21.
5. Sonmezer M, Oktay K. Fertility preservation in female patients. Hum Reprod Update. 2004;10(3):251–66.
6. Thomson AB et al. Late reproductive sequelae following treatment of childhood cancer and options for fertility preservation. Best Pract Res Clin Endocrinol Metab. 2002;16(2):311–34.
7. Wallace WH et al. Predicting age of ovarian failure after radiation to a field that includes the ovaries. Int J Radiat Oncol Biol Phys. 2005;62(3):738–44.
8. Wallace WH, Thomson AB, Kelsey TW. The radiosensitivity of the human oocyte. Hum Reprod. 2003;18(1):117–21.
9. Cağlar AA et al. Thyroid abnormalities in survivors of childhood cancer. J Clin Res Pediatr Endocrinol. 2014;6(3):144–51.
10. Meadows AT. Follow-up and care of childhood cancer survivors. Hosp Pract (Off Ed). 1991;26(2):99–102. 105-8.
11. Sklar C et al. Abnormalities of the thyroid in survivors of Hodgkin's disease: data from the Childhood Cancer Survivor Study. J Clin Endocrinol Metab. 2000;85(9):3227–32.
12. Knopman JM et al. Surviving childhood and reproductive-age malignancy: effects on fertility and future parenthood. Lancet Oncol. 2010;11(5):490–8.
13. Meirow D. Reproduction post-chemotherapy in young cancer patients. Mol Cell Endocrinol. 2000;169(1-2):123–31.
14. Green DM et al. Ovarian failure and reproductive outcomes after childhood cancer treatment: results from the Childhood Cancer Survivor Study. J Clin Oncol. 2009;27(14):2374–81.
15. Oktem O, Oktay K. Quantitative assessment of the impact of chemotherapy on ovarian follicle reserve and stromal function. Cancer. 2007;110(10):2222–9.
16. Gynecologic concerns in children and adolescents with cancer. Committee Opinion No. 607. Obstet Gynecol. 2014(124):403–8.

17. Lee SJ et al. American Society of Clinical Oncology recommendations on fertility preservation in cancer patients. J Clin Oncol. 2006;24(18):2917–31.

18. Hortobagyi GN et al. Immediate and long-term toxicity of adjuvant chemotherapy regimens containing doxorubicin in trials at M.D. Anderson Hospital and Tumor Institute. NCI Monogr. 1986;1:105–9.

19. Bines J, Oleske DM, Cobleigh MA. Ovarian function in premenopausal women treated with adjuvant chemotherapy for breast cancer. J Clin Oncol. 1996;14(5):1718–29.

20. Vatanen A et al. Ovarian function after allogeneic hematopoietic stem cell transplantation in childhood and adolescence. Eur J Endocrinol. 2014;170(2):211–8.

21. Bresters D et al. Ovarian insufficiency and pubertal development after hematopoietic stem cell transplantation in childhood. Pediatr Blood Cancer. 2014;61(11):2048–53.

22. Group CsO, editor. Long term follow-up guidelines for survivors of childhood, adolescent and young adult cancer. Version 3.0. Arcadia, CA: 2008.

23. Lunsford AJ et al. Antimullerian hormone as a measure of reproductive function in female childhood cancer survivors. Fertil Steril. 2014;101(1):227–31.

24. Knight PG, Glister C. TGF-beta superfamily members and ovarian follicle development. Reproduction. 2006;132(2):191–206.

25. Divasta AD, Gordon CM. Hormone replacement therapy and the adolescent. Curr Opin Obstet Gynecol. 2010;22(5):363–8.

26. Hershlag A, Rausch ME, Cohen M. Part 2: Ovarian failure in adolescent cancer survivors should be treated. J Pediatr Adolesc Gynecol. 2011;24(2):101–3.

27. DiVasta AD, Gordon CM. Hormone replacement therapy for the adolescent patient. Ann N Y Acad Sci. 2008;1135:204–11.

28. Kalantaridou SN et al. Impaired endothelial function in young women with premature ovarian failure: normalization with hormone therapy. J Clin Endocrinol Metab. 2004;89(8):3907–13.

29. Canonico M et al. Hormone therapy and venous thromboembolism among postmenopausal women: impact of the route of estrogen administration and progestogens: the ESTHER study. Circulation. 2007;115(7):840–5.

30. Scarabin PY et al. Differential association of oral and transdermal oestrogen-replacement therapy with venous thromboembolism risk. Lancet. 2003;362(9382):428–32.

31. Olie V, Canonico M, Scarabin PY. Risk of venous thrombosis with oral versus transdermal estrogen therapy among postmenopausal women. Curr Opin Hematol. 2010;17(5):457–63.

32. Welt CK. Primary ovarian insufficiency: a more accurate term for premature ovarian failure. Clin Endocrinol (Oxf). 2008;68(4):499–509.

33. Chow EJ et al. Timing of menarche among survivors of childhood acute lymphoblastic leukemia: a report from the Childhood Cancer Survivor Study. Pediatr Blood Cancer. 2008;50(4):854–8.

34. Metzger ML et al. Female reproductive health after childhood, adolescent, and young adult cancers: guidelines for the assessment and management of female reproductive complications. J Clin Oncol. 2013;31(9):1239–47.

35. Chow EJ et al. Decreased adult height in survivors of childhood acute lymphoblastic leukemia: a report from the Childhood Cancer Survivor Study. J Pediatr. 2007;150(4):370–5, 375.e1.

36. Groot-Loonen JJ et al. Shortened and diminished pubertal growth in boys and girls treated for acute lymphoblastic leukaemia. Acta Paediatr. 1996;85(9):1091–5.

37. Oostdijk W et al. Final height in central precocious puberty after long term treatment with a slow release GnRH agonist. Arch Dis Child. 1996; 75(4):292–7.

38. Bisharah M, Al-Fozan H, Tulandi T. A randomized trial of sublingual misoprostol for cervical priming before hysteroscopy. J Am Assoc Gynecol Laparosc. 2003;10(3):390–1.

39. Kuohung W et al. Laparoscopic oophoropexy prior to radiation for pediatric brain tumor and subsequent ovarian function. Hum Reprod. 2008; 23(1):117–21.

40. Bisharah M, Tulandi T. Laparoscopic preservation of ovarian function: an underused procedure. Am J Obstet Gynecol. 2003;188(2):367–70.

41. Anderson B et al. Ovarian transposition in cervical cancer. Gynecol Oncol. 1993;49(2):206–14.

42. Al-Badawi IA et al. Laparoscopic ovarian transposition before pelvic irradiation: a Saudi tertiary center experience. Int J Gynecol Cancer. 2010; 20(6):1082–6.

43. Schmidt KT et al. Risk of ovarian failure and fertility preserving methods in girls and adolescents with a malignant disease. BJOG. 2010;117(2):163–74.

44. Dolmans MM et al. Reimplantation of cryopreserved ovarian tissue from patients with acute lymphoblastic leukemia is potentially unsafe. Blood. 2010;116(16):2908–14.

45. Laufer MR et al. Ovarian tissue autologous transplantation to the upper extremity for girls receiving abdominal/pelvic radiation: 20-year follow-up of reproductive endocrine function. J Pediatr Adolesc Gynecol. 2010;23(2):107–10.

46. Oktay K et al. A technique for transplantation of ovarian cortical strips to the forearm. Fertil Steril. 2003;80(1):193–8.

47. Oktay K et al. Endocrine function and oocyte retrieval after autologous transplantation of ovarian cortical strips to the forearm. JAMA. 2001;286(12):1490–3.

48. Demeestere I et al. Live birth after autograft of ovarian tissue cryopreserved during childhood. Hum Reprod. 2015;30(9):2107–9.

49. Cobo A et al. Use of cryo-banked oocytes in an ovum donation programme: a prospective, randomized, controlled, clinical trial. Hum Reprod. 2010;25(9):2239–46.

50. von Wolff M et al. Ovarian stimulation to cryopreserve fertilized oocytes in cancer patients can be started in the luteal phase. Fertil Steril. 2009;92(4):1360–5.

Chapter 13
Pharmacological and Environmental Effects on Pubertal Development

Veronica Gomez-Lobo

Abbreviations

BMI   Body mass index
CPP   Central precocious puberty
DES   Diethylstilbestrol
ED   Endocrine disruptor
FSH   Follicle-stimulating hormone
LH   Luteinizing hormone

Introduction

During the first half of the twentieth century, there was noted a steep decline in the age of puberty and menarche in girls. It is thought that this decline most likely represents better nutrition as the western world developed. In the later part of the twentieth century, however,

V. Gomez-Lobo, M.D. (✉)
Washington Hospital Center/Children's National Medical Center,
Georgetown University, 110 Irving Street Rm 5B41, Washington,
DC 20010, USA
e-mail: veronica.gomez-lobo@medstar.net

© Springer International Publishing Switzerland 2016
H.L. Appelbaum (ed.), *Abnormal Female Puberty*,
DOI 10.1007/978-3-319-27225-2_13

there has been minimal decline in the age of menarche, but the age of thelarche appears to continue to decline [1]. In addition, the correlation of age of onset of breast development with menarche has decreased dramatically in the last decades such that the onset breast development is less predictive of the onset menarche than it once was [2, 3]. In addition, studies from Europe demonstrate that earlier menarche may be related to estradiol not stimulated by the hypothalamic–pituitary axis [3]. Given the relatively short period of time in which these later changes have taken place and the apparent peripheral cause of thelarche, it is likely that these changes are due to environmental or epigenetics (gene/environment interactions) rather than genetic alterations [1]. Some of these changes may be related to childhood obesity which is discussed in a previous chapter but exposures to medications and/or environmental agents may be involved in epidemiologic changes in obesity as well as puberty.

It is important to note that the changes in puberty can have significant impact on a girl's physical and emotional well-being. In addition, these changes may represent effects on the body which may in the future alter risks of other diseases such as cancers and metabolic syndromes [4]. This chapter will review possible pharmacologic and environmental effects on puberty.

Case Presentation

A mother presents with her 5-year-old daughter to the pediatrician's office stating that in the past few months she has noted that her daughter is developing breasts. She reports no pubic hair growth or vaginal bleeding. On review of systems, the child denies any headaches, seizures, abdominal pain, recent infections, or trauma and is not bothered by the changes in her body.

The mother reports that her daughter was born at term and has not had any illnesses. She is taking medication for attention deficit disorder and has no allergies.

She lives with both her parents and attends kindergarten in the local public school. There are no estrogenic medications in the house. Her mother had menarche at age 16 and does not remember when she began to develop breasts. She states that she emigrated from

India and is concerned that she may have been exposed to pesticides when pregnant with her daughter as she lived near some factories.

The child's physical exam is notable for a BMI and height in the 95 % for age. She has no skin abnormalities or thyromegaly. Heart, lung, and abdominal exam are normal. Her breasts are Tanner 2 by palpation, and her pubic hair is Tanner 1. Genital exam reveals normal prepubertal female genitalia without clitoromegaly and a crescentic shaped hymen that is patent without signs of estrogenization. There is no discharge or lesions noted.

Laboratory analysis reveals slightly elevated luteinizing hormone (LH) and follicle-stimulating hormone (FSH), and estradiol for a prepubertal girl. A pelvic ultrasound reveals prepubertal appearing uterus and ovaries without masses. Bone age is slightly advanced compared to chronologic age.

Discussion

Effects of Puberty Disruptors

Endocrine disruptors (ED) are thought to be environmental chemicals, dietary supplements, and/or medications which interfere with or alter the body's endocrine system. Some endocrine disruptors may act by mimicking the effects of natural hormones and others may bind receptors and block their actions. In addition, they may interfere with the production, transport, metabolism, and/or excretion of naturally occurring hormones [4]. Furthermore, some of the effects of EDs may be transmitted to future generations through germ line epigenetic modifications [5].

Factors regulating the onset of puberty are poorly understood thus elucidating which substances function as endocrine disruptors is difficult. There is convincing evidence that EDs affect pubertal timing in animals but the data in humans has been more difficult to interpret due to the many confounders inherent to the epidemiologic research [3]. These include the size of the sample population, the choice of end points (menarche vs. thelarche), the choice of possible confounders, etc. [6] Thus at this time, there is an incomplete understanding of which agents actually function as endocrine disruptors in large populations and the mechanism of action for their effects.

Timing and Amount of Exposure

Often populations are exposed to mixtures of agents, and it is not easy to tease out the effect of each agent. Some combinations of substances, for example, may have additive or even synergistic effects. In addition, the quantity of exposure is often difficult to ascertain. Furthermore, in the case of pharmacologic exposures, it may be difficult to interpret whether the medication or the underlying condition or the combination are effecting puberty. For many of these exposures, there may be a critical window of susceptibility, and that window of exposure may be separated from the effect by a long period of time, making it difficult to correlate these two events. For example, in utero occurrences may have effects on puberty as evidenced by the fact that children who are born small for gestational age are at risk of earlier onset of pubertal development and menarche [7]. Other periods of susceptibility may include the neonatal and prepubertal times. Thus, several of the epidemiologic studies evaluating environmental exposures have looked at the offspring of women exposed at work (occupational) or in areas with accidental exposure during pregnancy and/or during the period of breastfeeding. Other studies have evaluated children who may have been exposed during the juvenile or pubertal period.

Obesity

In the past four decades, there has been a sharp increase in childhood obesity both in developed and developing nations which has been attributed to an imbalance between dietary intake and caloric expenditure [1]. Experts, however, have more recently highlighted other possible contributing factors such as changes in microbiotic flora, epigenetic modifications, increasing maternal age, changes in the intrauterine environment as well as possible exposure to endocrine disrupting and other pharmacologic agents [8]. Many, though not all, endocrine disruptors may affect puberty through effects on body mass and obesity [1]. These substances mostly contribute to obesity by promoting either the number or size of adipocytes but may also have indirect effects by promoting changes in basal metabolic rate and altering hormonal control of appetite and satiety [1]. In mice, for example, low doses of exposure to diethylstilbestrol (DES) in utero or early life caused an increase in body weight as well as earlier puberty [9]. There are several potential ways in which body fat may influence the onset of puberty: adipokines such as leptin may have a direct effect, aromatase action in adipocytes may increase conversion of androgens to estrogen, and adipose tissue can influence insulin resistance which lowers sex hormone globulin and thus may lead to greater bioavailability of sex steroids [1].

Examples of Possible Puberty Disruptors

Neuromodulators: Medications to Treat Psychiatric Illness and Seizures

Several neuromodulators have been mentioned as possible disruptors of puberty but have not been well studied. Valproic acid, an antiepileptic, has been noted to induce obesity, hyperandrogenism, menstrual disorders, polycystic ovary syndrome, hyperinsulinism, changes in gonadotropic, sex and thyroid hormones as well as pubertal development and impaired skeletal growth [10]. On the other hand, a controlled study in children with attention deficit hyperactivity disorder (ADHD) between ages 10 and 14 revealed a trend for stimulant-associated delayed puberty [11].

Nutritional Supplements and Vitamins

Nutritional supplements as well as excess or lack of certain nutrients may have endocrine disrupting effects on puberty. A case control prospective study in Columbia did reveal that girls with vitamin D deficiency had earlier menarche when compared to their non-deficient counterparts, and these differences could not be accounted for by body mass index differences alone [12]. Lignans and flavonols are phytoestrogens which are found in fruits, grains, and vegetables and are found in high concentrations in the Western diet [13]. In a study in the United States, the highest flavonol intake was associated with later breast development [13]. A study of infant feeding exposure to soy (another phytoestrogen) suggested that earlier menarche events occurred more frequently in the early soy group, as compared to other feeding groups [14]. On the other hand, a cross-sectional study of adolescent soy food consumption did not reveal an association between soy intake and age of menarche [15]. These different findings may be due to the different time of exposure (possibly due to a window of susceptibility) as well as the study methods.

Environmental Exposures

Several agents that are encountered in the environment have been described as endocrine disruptors [3, 4]. Exposure to these agents can result from chronic low-dose exposures in food contamination, inhalation of contaminated dust, or occupational exposures [16]. Most of the studies regarding the effect of particular agents reviewed large industrial accidental exposure and given the inherent issues with epidemiologic studies as described above there are some conflicting reports regarding their effects. The flame retardant polybrominated biphenyl (PBB), the coolant polychlorinated biphenyl (PCB) (both of which are banned in the United States), the pesticide dichlorodiphenyltrichloroethane (DDT) and its derivative dichlorodiphenyltrichloroethane (DDE) have been described as estrogenic or antiandrogenic in animal studies and have been noted in several cohorts to be associated with early thelarche and some with early menarche [5, 17]. Though many of these agents have been banned from most Western countries, a study in girls in Belgium who were adopted from endemic areas reveals that they had earlier puberty than non-adopted girls. This data, however, does not exclude the possibility that these girls may have had intrauterine growth restriction with subsequent catch up upon migration which may cause precocious puberty [17]. Phthalates are present in food packaging materials and are ubiquitous in the environment. In a case control study in Puerto Rico, girls with premature thelarche were more likely to have detectable levels and higher concentrations of phthalates than in controls, though this study has been disputed [6]. Biphenol A (BPA) is found in plastics and cans and is thought to have estrogenic effects. Exposure to BPA (evaluated by urinary levels) in 9 year olds of both sexes reveal a correlation with adiposity in these children and disturbed puberty is noted in exposed animals [17]. Prenatal and postpartum exposure to dioxins (by-products of industrial processes), on the other hand, have been shown in two studies to cause a delay in thelarche [6, 17]. Given these findings, it is important that we continue to monitor the possible endocrine effects of frequently encountered environmental substances.

Other Agents

When children have chronic illnesses which require medications, it is difficult to assess whether early or delayed puberty are effects of the underlying condition or the medications that treat these. Many childhood illnesses are treated with long-term corticosteroids. These have effects on growth and skeletal muscle [18–20]. Data on pubertal development in adolescents after renal transplantation as well as in children with juvenile idiopathic arthritis suggests that puberty may be delayed in children with these conditions [18, 20]. Steroid use, however, correlated with delayed puberty only in boys but not in girls with juvenile arthritis [16]. In children with kidney transplants, the delayed puberty was noted to be mostly due to poor graft function and interval since transplant rather than medications [20].

It should be noted that survival rates from childhood cancers have improved dramatically in the past few decades. In addition, other conditions such as systemic lupus erythematous are treated with steroids as well as cytotoxic agents. Several chemotherapeutic agents and radiation have been noted to cause premature ovarian failure which may prevent a child from entering or completing pubertal development. Current recommendations are that patients and families be counseled regarding the possible loss of fertility [21].

Management and Outcome

The girl presented in the case above has early thelarche which may be due to central precocious puberty. The causes of central precocious puberty include central nervous system tumors, trauma, and lesions but most often is idiopathic. Peripheral precocious puberty may be due to estrogen production due to tumor, spontaneous follicular development, or McCune–Albright syndrome. There can also be pubertal development in girls treated with, or inadvertently taking, estrogen. In this case, there are no obvious inciting factors aside from obesity. Her mother is concerned that she may have had exposures which may influence her daughter's pubertal development. The family was counseled that environmental exposures to pesticides as well as obesity, certain medications as well as growth restriction in utero or early childhood may be linked to earlier puberty. They were further counseled about proper diet and exercise for a child her age. She was referred to a pediatric endocrinologist to monitor her pubertal development.

Clinical Pearls/Pitfalls

1. Recent epidemiologic changes have been noted in the onset and progress of puberty in girls in the Western world.
2. Several agents have been identified as possible endocrine disruptors including environmental chemicals, nutritional supplements as well as medications, but the data regarding their effects are far from conclusive.
3. Given the importance of puberty for individuals as well as the possible public health effects of its alterations, it is important that we continue to monitor changes in populations and attempt to elucidate possible causal agents and the mechanism by which they influence puberty.

References

1. Biro FM, Greenspan LC, Galvez MP. Puberty in girls in the 21st century. J Pediatr Adolesc Gynecol. 2012;25(5):289–94. PMID 22841372.
2. Biro FM, Huang B, Crawford PB, et al. Pubertal correlates in black and white girls. J Pediatr. 2006;148(2):234–40. PMID: 16492435.
3. Walvoord EC. The timing of puberty: is it changing? Does it matter? J Adolesc Health. 2010;47(5):433–9. PMDI 20970077.
4. Biro FM, Deardorff J. Identifying opportunities for cancer prevention during preadolescence and adolescence: puberty as a window of susceptibility. J Adolesc Health. 2013;52(6):808. PMDI 23601607.
5. Diamanti-Kandarakis E, Bourguignon JP, Giudice LC, et al. Endocrine-disrupting chemicals: An endocrine society scientific statement. Endocr Rev. 2009;30(4):293–342. PMDI 19502515.
6. Den Hond E, Schoeters G. Endocrine disrupters and human puberty. Int J Androl. 2006;29(1):264–71. PMID:16466548.
7. Verkauskiene R, Petraitiene I, Albertsson WK. Puberty in children born small for gestational age. Horm Res Paediatr. 2013;80(2):69–77. PMDI 23899516.
8. McAllister EJ, Dhurandhar NV, Keith SW, et al. Ten putative contributors to the obesity epidemic. Crit Rev Food Sci Nutr. 2009;49(10):868–913. PMID 19960394.
9. Newbold RR, Padilla-Banks E, Snyder RJ, et al. Developmental exposure to estrogenic compounds and obesity. Birth Defects Res A Clin Mol Teratol. 2005;73(7):478–80. PMID 15959888.
10. Verrotti A, Greco R, Latini G, Chiarelli F. Endocrine and metabolic changes in epileptic patients receiving valproic acid. J Pediatr Endocrinol Metab. 2005;18(5):423–30. PMID 15921170.
11. Greenfield B, Hechtman L, Stehli A, Wigal T. Sexual maturation among youth with ADHD and the impact of stimulant medication. Eur Child Adolesc Psychiatry. 2014;23(9):835–9. PMDI 24488239.
12. Chew A, Harris SS. Does vitamin D affect timing of menarche? Nutr Rev. 2013;71(3):189–93. PMDI 23452286.
13. Mervish NA, Gardiner EW, Galvez MP, et al. Dietary flavonol intake is associated with age of puberty in a longitudinal cohort of girls. Nutr Res. 2013;33(7):534–42. PMDI 23827127.
14. Adgent MA, Daniels JL, Rogan WJ, et al. Early-life exposure and age at menarche. Paediatr Perinat Epidemiol. 2012;26(2):163–75. PMDI 22324503.
15. Segovia-Siapco G, Pribis P, Messina M, et al. Is soy intake related to age at onset of menarche? A cross-sectional study of adolescents with a wide range of soy food consumption. Nutr J. 2014;13:54. PMDI 2488955.
16. Frye CA, Bo E, Calamandrei G, et al. Endocrine disrupters: a review of some sources, effects, and mechanism of actions on behaviour and neuroendocrine systems. J Neuroendocrinol. 2012;24(1):144–59. PMDI 21951193.

17. Bourguignon JP, Franssen D, Gerard A, et al. Early neuroendocrine disruption in hypothalamus and hippocampus: developmental effects including female sexual maturation and implications for endocrine disrupting chemical screening. J Neuroendocrinol. 2013;25(11):1079–87. PMDI 24028442.

18. El Badr D, Rostom S, Bouaddi I, et al. Sexual maturation in Moroccan patients with juvenile idiopathic arthritis. Rheumatol Int. 2014;34(5):665–8. PMDI 23553519.

19. Ghanem ME, Eman ME, Albaghdady LA, et al. Effect of childhood kidney transplantation on puberty. Fertil Steril. 2010;94(6):2248–52. PMID 20149362.

20. Tainio J, Qvist E, Vehmas R, et al. Pubertal development is normal in adolescents after renal transplantation in childhood. Transplantation. 2011;92(4):404–9. PMID 21709603.

21. Blumenfeld Z. Chemotherapy and fertility. Best Pract Res Clin Obstet Gynaecol. 2012;26(3):379–90. PMID 22281514.

Index

A

Abnormal androgen metabolism
  amenorrhea
    baseline laboratory tests, 118
    delayed puberty/absent
      menses, 118
    management, 119, 122
    metformin, 121
    oligomenorrhea, 121
    outcome, 120, 122
    physical examination,
      118, 120
    sex hormone production, 119
  axillary and pubic hair, 117
    laboratory tests, 115
    management, 116
    outcome, 117
    physical examination, 115
    precocious pubarche and
      thelarche, 115, 116
  hypertension, 120
    baseline laboratory tests, 118
    delayed puberty/absent
      menses, 118
    management, 119
    outcome, 120
    physical examination, 118
    sex hormone production, 119
  irregular periods
    laboratory tests, 111
    management, 113, 114
    non-ovulatory menstrual
      pattern, 111
    outcome, 114
    patient's lab data, 112
    physical examination, 111
Acid labile subunit (ALS), 50
Amenorrhea, 2, 120, 122
  baseline laboratory tests, 118
  delayed puberty/absent
    menses, 118
  management, 119, 122
  metformin, 121
  oligomenorrhea, 121
  outcome, 120, 122
  physical examination, 118, 120
  sex hormone production, 119
American College of Sports
    Medicine (ACSM), 177
Androgen insensitivity (AIS)
  clinical presentation, 11
  DSDs, 12
  excess androgen hormone
    production, 12
  gonadectomy, 14
  management, 16–17

© Springer International Publishing Switzerland 2016
H.L. Appelbaum (ed.), *Abnormal Female Puberty*,
DOI 10.1007/978-3-319-27225-2

Androgen insensitivity (AIS) (*cont.*)
    nonsurgical and surgical
        techniques, 15
    optimal clinical management,
        14, 16
    outcomes, 17
    qualitative mutation, 13
    receptor impairment, 13
    Wolffiann system, 15, 16
    X chromosome, 13
Anorexia nervosa, 172
    BMI, 152
    diagnosis, 156–157
        ARFID, 160–161
        bulimia nervosa, 160
        EDNOS, 159–160
        pre- and peri-pubertal
            patients, 158–159
        weight gain/body image
            distortion, 157–158
    management
        electrolyte/cardiac
            abnormalities, 169–170
        growth curve, 153, 168
        in-patient settings, 171
        medical, nutritional, and
            psychological factors,
            167–169
        out-patient settings, 169
        standard interpersonal
            therapy, 170–171
    medical complications
        cardiovascular
            abnormalities, 163
        delayed menarche, 164–166
        energy-deficient state,
            163–164
        gastrointestinal
            abnormalities, 163
        hematologic
            abnormalities, 163
        malnutrition, 162
        metabolic abnormalities,
            162–163
        neurologic abnormalities, 163
        osteopenia/osteoporosis,
            166–167
    outcome, 171
    physical examination, 155
    protein calorie malnutrition, 152
    treatment, 155
Anti-mullerian hormone (AMH), 78
Ataxia telangiectasia (AT), 74
Avoidant-Restrictive Food Intake
        Disorder (ARFID),
        160–161

B
Body mass index (BMI), 152

C
Celiac disease (CD), 220
    bloating and frequent
        flatulence, 210
    clinical and epidemiological
        studies, 211
    diagnosis, 213–216
    epidemiology, 212, 213
    fertility, 211
    genetics, 212, 213
    GFD, 212
    irregular menstrual cycle, 211
    management, 216–219
    outcomes, 220
    pathology, 210
    physical examination, 209
    poor weight gain and short
        stature, 208
    serum laboratory tests, 209
Constitutional delay of growth and
        puberty (CDGP), 50, 63
    breast budding, 48, 49
    diagnosis
        assessment, 58–59
        bone age radiograph, 57
        GnRH stimulation testing,
            57–58
        initial laboratory evaluation,
            56–57
    estrogen, 61
    evaluation
        birth history, 52

delayed puberty, 52–53
growth curve, 54–56
MPH, 54–55
Turner syndrome, 51–52
genetic analysis
ALS, 50
heterozygous novel
missense variant, 49
pericentrometeric
region, 50
X-linked and autosomal
recessive forms, 49
hypogonadotrophic
hypogonadism, 51
lack of menarche, 48, 49
long-term prognosis
adult height and fertility,
61, 62
SDS, 62
outcome, 62, 63
oxandrolone
dose-related side effects, 60
female populations, 60
growth plate maturation,
58–59
growth velocity, 60
Turner syndrome, 60
therapeutic options, 58
Cryopreservation
autotransplantation, 255
fertility preservation, 254
ovarian cortex, 254
prepubertal children, 255

D
Delayed puberty. *See* Endocrine
disorders
Dual energy X-ray absorptiometry
(DXA) scan, 81
Dysgerminoma, 228

E
Eating disorder not otherwise
specified (EDNOS), 156,
157, 160–161

Endocrine disorders
hyperprolactinemia, 104
management, 103
menstrual irregularity, 101
outcome, 103
physical examination, 101
prolactin, 102
hypothyroidism, 97
delayed and precocious
puberty, 96
irregular menses, 95
management, 97
outcome, 97
overactive and underactive
thyroid conditions, 96
physical examination, 95
thyroid studies, 95
panhypopituitarism, 101
laboratory evaluation, 98
lack of gonadotropin, 98, 99
management, 99, 100
outcome, 100
physical examination, 98
vaginal bleeding, 97
POI, 94
diagnosis, 91
gonadotropins, 91
laboratory testing, 90
management, 92–94
maternal menarche, 89
outcome, 94
physical examination, 90
primary amenorrhea, 90
X-chromosome defect, 92
Endocrine disruptors (ED), 41
environmental chemicals, 40
laboratory testing, 39
management, 40, 41
outcome, 41
pharmacological effects, 263
vaginal discharge/bleeding, 39

G
Gonadotropin-dependent,
precocious puberty
(GDPP), 27

I
Imperforate hymen
  clinical presentation, 7, 8
  management, 10–11
  obstructive reproductive
      anomaly, 7
  outcomes, 11
  pelvic MRI, 7, 9
  transverse vaginal septum, 9

M
Mayer–Rokitansky–Küster–Hauser
    (MRKH), 4
Mid-parental height (MPH), 54–55
Müllerian agenesis
  abnormal puberty, 3
  clinical presentation, 2–3
  management, 5–6
  MRKH, 4
  outcome, 6
  pelvic ultrasound, 3, 4
Müllerian duct anomalies (MDA), 4

N
Neuromodulators, 265

O
Obesity
  adolescence
    environmental factors, 134
    food consumption, 132
    genetic and environmental
        factors, 135
    insulin resistance, 136
    intermediate factors, 140
    large-scale study, 135, 136
    leptin, 138–140
    management, 144
    menstrual irregularities,
        142, 143
    multifactorial disease, 132
    outcome, 145

    physical activity, 134
    physiology, 137, 138
    short- and long-term
        implications, 141, 142
    weight status, 136, 137
  in childhood
    definition, 130
    environmental factors, 134
    genetic and environmental
        factors, 135
    home and school
        environments, 134
    insulin resistance, 136
    intermediate factors, 140
    large-scale study,
        135, 136
    leptin, 138–140
    management, 144
    menstrual irregularities,
        142, 143
    multifactorial disease, 132
    outcome, 145
    physical activity, 134
    physiology, 137, 138
    prevalence, 130
    prevention and treatment, 130
    short- and long-term
        implications, 141, 142
    weight status, 136, 137
  maternal menarche, 129
  physical examination, 129
Ovarian neoplasms, 236
  abdominal pain
    acne and coarse hair, 225
    benign and malignant
        ovarian neoplasms, 226
    in childhood and
        adolescence, 226
    epithelial ovarian
        tumors, 233
    germ cell tumors, 228–231
    leukemia/lymphoma, 233
    normal fertility potential, 234
    ovarian torsion, 227
    physical examination, 225

small cell carcinoma, 233
stromal tumors, 231, 232
transvaginal sonography,
226–227
vaccination schedule, 225
management, 235
outcome, 235

P
Pharmacological effects, 262,
263, 268
accidental exposure, 264
chemotherapeutic agents and
radiation, 267
chronic illnesses, 267
cytotoxic agents, 267
endocrine disruptors, 263
environmental exposures,
266, 267
management and outcome, 268
neuromodulators, 265
nutritional supplements, 265
obesity, 264, 265
vaginal bleeding
laboratory analysis, 263
medication, 262
physical examination, 263
vitamins, 265, 266
Post-menarche, 256
Precocious puberty, 251, 252, 256
brain tumor, 30
bone age X-ray, 26
endocrinological
evaluation, 25
environmental exposures, 26
GDPP, 27
hypothalamic hamartomas, 27
imaging studies, 28
management, 29
neurofibromatosis type 1, 28
outcome, 30
premature adrenarche, 27
prior growth curves, 25
pubertal development, 26

radiation, 250
causes, 24
classifications, 25
endocrine disruptors, 41
environmental chemicals, 40
laboratory testing, 39
management, 40, 41
outcome, 41
vaginal discharge/bleeding, 39
exogenous hormones, 39
laboratory testing, 38
management, 38
maternal menarche, 37
outcome, 38
Tanner stage 1, 37
Tanner stage 3, 37
head trauma, 36
laboratory testing, 35
management, 36
outcome, 36
severe automobile
accident, 34
Tanner stage 3, 35
TBI, 35
ovarian cyst, 34
abdominal pain/distention, 32
acne/adult body odors,
30, 31
differential diagnosis, 32
growth acceleration, 31
laboratory testing, 31
management, 33
outcome, 34
transabdominal pelvic
ultrasound, 33
physical examination, 250
premature activation, 250
Premature ovarian failure (POF), 83
anti-adrenal antibody titers,
76, 77
AT, 74
ataxia telangiectasia, 71
autoimmune lymphocytic
oophoritis, 76
cerebral palsy, 71

Premature ovarian failure
        (POF) (cont.)
    diagnostic evaluation
        AMH, 79
        clinical presentation, 78
        DXA scan, 81
        estrogen replacement, 79
        non-aromatizable anabolic
                steroid, 80
        peak bone density, 80
        subspecialist referral, 80
    etiology and timing, 77
    galactosemia, 77
    hypergonadotropic
                hypogonadism, 71
    outcomes, 81, 82
    polymorphisms and mutations, 74
    sex chromosomes, 72
    STAG3 expression, 74
    Turner syndrome
        amniocentesis, 68
        cardinal features, 75
        gonadal dysgenesis, 74
        growth failure, 70
        physical examination, 70
        primordial germ cells, 75
Premenarche
    autotransplantation, 255
    fertility preservation, 254
    ovarian cortex, 254
    prepubertal children, 255
Primary amenorrhea, 249, 250
    advantages, 248
    chemotherapy regimen,
                244, 245
    Hodgkin disease, 243
    hypothyroidism, 244
    lab tests, 243
    management, 246–248
    median lethal dose, 244
    outcome, 249
    physical examination, 243
    POF, 244
    severe gonadal damage, 245
    transdermal/oral routes, 249

Primary ovarian insufficiency
        (POI), 94
    diagnosis, 91
    gonadotropins, 91
    laboratory testing, 90
    management, 92–94
    maternal menarche, 89
    outcome, 94
    physical examination, 90
    primary amenorrhea, 90
    X-chromosome defect, 92

S
Secondary amenorrhea, 197, 198
    adverse health outcomes,
                183, 184
    laboratory testing, 177
    management
        bone health assessment, 181,
                182, 188, 190
        energy availability, 178–180,
                186, 187
        medical history, 185
        menstrual abnormalities,
                176, 187, 188
        physical examination, 185
        prevention, 196
        screening, 195, 196
        treatment, 191–193
        triad, 194
    menstrual function, 180, 181
    outcome, 197
    physical activity, 177
    physical examination, 176
Sertoli–Leydig tumors, 232
Stromal antigen 3 (STAG3), 74

T
Traumatic brain injury (TBI), 35

U
Ultrasound, 12, 33, 91

V
Valsalva maneuvering, 7, 9
Vitamins
    adolescent girls, 192
    amenorrhea, 120
    panhypopituitarism, 98
    pharmacological effects, 265, 266

POF, 81
primary amenorrhea, 11

X
X chromosome, 13, 52, 72, 75

Printed in the United States
By Bookmasters